KEY CLINICAL TRIALS IN BPH

Editors:
Darracott Vaughan and Georg Bartsch

Series Editors:
Peter Boyle and Mike Wyllie

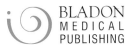

BLADON
MEDICAL
PUBLISHING

| CONTENTS | Page |

KEY
CLINICAL
TRIALS IN
BPH

© 2002 Bladon Medical Publishing
12 New Street, Chipping Norton, Oxfordshire
OX7 5LJ, UK

First published 2002

Always refer to the manufacturer's Prescribing
Information before prescribing drugs cited in this
book.

British Library Cataloguing in Publication Data.
A catalogue record for this title is available from the
British Library

ISBN 1-904218-03-2

D Vaughan, G Bartsch, P Boyle and M Wyllie
Key Clinical Trials in BPH

Project Editor: Fiona Swingland

Design and production:
Design Online Ltd, Oxford

Printed by
Grafiche IGC S.R.L.,
25128 Brescia, Zona Industriale,
Via A. Grandi, 29, Italy

Distributed by
Plymbridge Distributors Ltd, Estover Road,
Plymouth PL6 7PY, UK

Abbreviations

a	approximately
ACE	angiotensin-converting enzyme
AEs	adverse events
AUA	American Urological Association
AUA-SS	American Urological Association Symptom Score
AUA-BS	American Urological Association Bother Score
AUR	acute urinary retention
b.i.d.	twice daily dosing
BII	BPH Impact Index
BPH	benign prostatic hyperplasia
BP	blood pressure
DRE	digital rectal examination
DBP	diastolic blood pressure
EAU	European Association of Urology
GITS	Gastrointestinal Therapeutic System
GP	general practitioner
HR	heart rate
HRQL	health related quality of life
IIEF	International Index of Erectile Function
IPSS	International Prostate Symptom Score
LHRH	luteinising hormone-releasing hormone
LUTS	lower urinary tract symptoms
n	number (of patients)
o.d.	once daily dosing
PFR	peak flow rate
PVR	post void residual urine volume
QoL	quality of life
SBP	systolic blood pressure
t.i.d.	three times daily dosing

Key to study schematics:

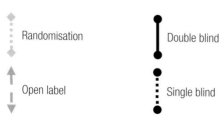

Randomisation

Open label

Double blind

Single blind

Over the last three decades the medical management of the lower urinary tract symptoms (LUTS) in BPH patients has evolved considerably from being the exclusive domain of the urological surgeon. Although surgery still has an important role to play the use of drugs in the hands of specialists and primary care physicians has increased dramatically. A major stimulus for this was the pioneering work of Marco Caine in a carefully controlled clinical setting using objective clinical endpoints: in other words a clinical trial that was key to our attitude to patient management.

Contained within this slim volume are some of the other Key Clinical Trials that have influenced our thinking in the treatment of LUTS. In an attempt to understand the potential significance, a critique of the studies' strengths and weaknesses is included well as a diagrammatic summary of the trial design and key result(s). Most of the studies have appeared in peer group reviewed journals and the data from each can be recycled in many different papers. For this reason, few of the trials are listed as single journal reference and often in fact a list of relevant citations is given. The editors have adopted the philosophy that a study does not have to be any or all of "gold standard", "placebo-controlled", "randomised", "adequately powered" "regulatory-standard", "pivotal" or "meta-analysis" to merit inclusion. The trial has merely to satisfy the criterion that it has or will profoundly influence the way BPH patients are managed.

In many cases it would have been possible to select several clinical trials. For example combination studies have now been completed with finasteride and alfuzosin, doxazosin and terazosin. However, an analysis of only one of these, the first involving terazosin, serves as a model of all others and is therefore used for illustrative purposes. Trial selection was the subject of considerable debate and to ensure independence those included in this volume of Key Clinical Trials were nominated by Darracott Vaughan and Georg Bartsch.

Peter Boyle and Mike Wyllie

STUDY DESCRIPTOR

The trial that laid down the foundation for the use of drugs in managing BPH/LUTS: Phenoxybenzamine in the treatment of benign prostatic obstruction.

KEY TRIAL REFERENCES

MAJOR PUBLICATION:
Caine M, Perlberg S, Meretyk S. A placebo controlled, double-blind study of the effect of phenoxybenzamine in benign prostatic obstruction. Br J Urol 50:551-554, 1978.

ORIGINAL ABSTRACT: Caine M. BAUS: 1978

OTHER IMPORTANT PUBLICATIONS:
Caine M, Perlberg S, Shapiro A. Phenoxybenzamine for benign prostatic obstruction: Review of 200 cases. Urology 17(6):542-546, 1981.

Caine M. Clinical experience with alpha-adrenoreceptor antagonists in benign prostatic hypertrophy. Fed Proc 45(11):2604-2608, 1986.

STUDY FUNDING:

IMPORTANCE OF STUDY

This clinical trial forms the foundation for all drugs used in the management of BPH. It is considered to be the definitive study showing the benefits of α-blockade in BPH patients.

Study Design

Randomised, double-blind, placebo-controlled study. n=50.
Patients were randomised to receive either phenoxybenzamine 10 mg b.i.d. (n=24)
or placebo (n=26) for 14 days treatment.

Outcome measures:
PFR, mean flow rate, PVR urine, urethral pressure and were assessed at baseline and
at the end of the study. Changes in diurnal and nocturnal micturition frequencies
were also recorded.

Inclusion criteria: BPH patients attending outpatient clinic.

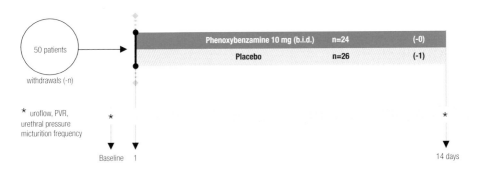

KEY RESULTS

- Phenoxybenzamine produced highly significant improvements in PFR (87.5%) compared to placebo (18.5%). Similarly there were significant improvements in mean flow rate (phenoxybenzamine 81.9% and placebo 30.4%).

- However, there was no difference in PVR urine between the 2 treatment groups.

- Daytime micturition frequency (ability to hold urine 1 hour or more longer) was improved in 54% of phenoxybenzamine patients compared to 20% with placebo. Nocturnal frequency (necessity to pass urine one or more less times in the night) was also improved with phenoxybenzamine (67% vs 32% placebo).

- Urethral pressure recordings confirmed that there was a reduction in the closure pressure in the prostatic segment of the urethra with phenoxybenzamine treatment.

- Side effects were reported in 46% of phenoxybenzamine patients (commonly tiredness or slight dizziness) compared to 4% (1 patient) with placebo.

Clinical benefit of the α-blocker phenoxybenzamine, in the treatment of symptomatic BPH following treatment for 2 weeks

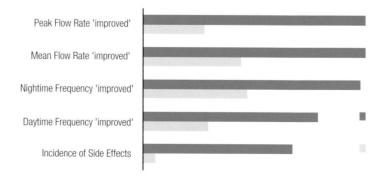

Conclusions from Original Reports

Phenoxybenzamine is of practical value in the symptomatic treatment of benign prostatic obstruction.

The reduction in intraurethral pressure in the region of the prostate corresponds well to the improvement in urinary flow rate in phenoxybenzamine treated patients.

Popular Citation: not applicable

Strengths

A placebo-controlled study using validated urodynamic endpoints (mean flow rate and residual urine) in a reasonably sized patient population.

Weaknesses

By today's standards, this clinical trial design (no symptom scoring) and powering would be considered to be somewhat limited. However, this study is representative of subsequent larger studies.

Relevance

The results of this trial are consistent with the clinical benefit seen with the newer generation of α-blockers, in the treatment of lower urinary tract symptoms (LUTS) in BPH patients. However, due to problems with patient compliance, phenoxybenzamine is no longer widely used.

One of the first carefully controlled studies looking at the overall therapeutic benefit of an alpha-blocker: Terazosin in the management of the symptoms associated with benign prostatic hyperplasia.

KEY TRIAL REFERENCES

MAJOR PUBLICATION:
Lepor H, Auerbach S et al. A randomised, placebo-controlled multicentre study of the efficacy and safety of terazosin in the treatment of benign prostatic hyperplasia. J Urol 148:1467-1474, 1992.

ORIGINAL ABSTRACT: not published at AUA or EAU

OTHER IMPORTANT PUBLICATIONS:
Lepor H. Long-term efficacy and safety of terazosin in patients with benign prostatic hyperplasia. Terazosin Research Group. Urology 45(3):406-413, 1995.

Boyle P, Robinson C et al. Meta-analysis of randomised trials of Terazosin in the treatment of benign prostatic hyperplasia. Urology 58(5): 717-722, 2001.

STUDY FUNDING: Abbott Laboratories

IMPORTANCE OF STUDY

One of the first carefully controlled clinical trials showing unequivocally the clinical benefit of an α-blocker for the treatment of BPH.
This study became the benchmark for the pivotal studies required by the FDA and other regulatory authorities for drug registration.
The clinical profile of terazosin was later confirmed by meta-analysis.

Study Design

Randomised, double-blind, placebo-controlled, multicentre study. n=285.
421 patients entered the single-blind, placebo lead-in phase of 4 weeks. Qualifying patients (n=285) entered a 12-week treatment period and were randomised in a double-blind fashion to receive either terazosin (2, 5 or 10mg o.d.) or placebo. Terazosin doses were titrated during a dose escalation period of up to 4 weeks (depending on the dose). Patients then continued on their assigned dose for a minimum of 8 weeks.

Outcome measures:
Boyarsky symptom scores (9 symptoms, scored 0-3), uroflow (PFR, mean flow rate) and BP were assessed at baseline, 2, 4, 6, 8, 10, 12, 14 and 16 weeks.
Patient symptom diaries and side effects (spontaneous reporting).

Inclusion criteria:
50-75 years, Boyarsky ≥ 1 on 2 or more of the obstructive symptom subscores. PFR 5-12ml/s, PVR urine ≤ 200ml, DBP < 115mmHg.

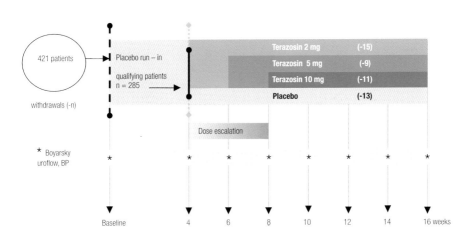

Key Results

- Boyarsky symptom scores (obstructive, irritative and total) were significantly improved versus placebo, for all terazosin treatment groups. The percentage change in total Boyarsky symptom score (intention to treat analysis) for the placebo, 2mg, 5mg and 10mg groups were 23%, 32%, 32% and 44% respectively. Similarly, the percentage of patients experiencing greater than 30% improvement in total symptom scores were 40%, 51%, 51% and 69%.

- PFR and mean flow rates were both significantly improved in the 10mg terazosin group. The percentage improvements in PFR (intention to treat analysis) for the placebo, 2mg, 5mg and 10mg groups were 10%, 24%, 19% and 29% respectively.

- Adverse events in all groups were minor and reversible. Although there were higher frequencies of asthenia, 'flu syndrome and dizziness reported in the terazosin treatment groups, these did not reach statistical significance compared to placebo. The proportion of patients withdrawing due to adverse events from the terazosin groups was similar to placebo.

- The mean decrease in DBP was significantly greater in the 5mg and 10mg terazosin groups (compared to placebo), but the change in SBP for these patients was not.

Short-term efficacy of terazosin for the treatment of symtomatic BPH. Changes in efficacy outcomes from baseline to final visit compared to placebo (minimum of 8 weeks treatment steady dose)

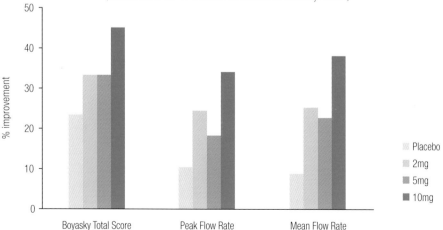

Conclusions from Original Reports

This study unequivocally supports the short-term efficacy and safety of terazosin for the treatment of symptomatic BPH.

Improvements in both symptom score and urinary flow rates did not reach a plateau within the dose range evaluated in this study, suggesting that further improvements in efficacy may be achieved at doses exceeding 10mg.

Popular Citation: not applicable

Strengths

A well designed, placebo-controlled study in a large number of patients.

Weaknesses

The Boyarsky scoring system used in this study has been replaced by the AUA symptom score and the IPSS.

The original study was only over 3 months, however it was subsequently extended.

Relevance

This study is entirely predictive of the clinical profile of terazosin in the hands of the specialist and the primary care physician. This profile has been subsequently confirmed by meta-analysis of all terazosin studies.

This study is the fore-runner of many similar studies on other α-blockers in the management of BPH.

A clinical trials design standard, based on an examination of the long-term effects of an alpha-blocker in a community setting: Terazosin in the long-term treatment of symptomatic benign prostatic hyperplasia.

KEY TRIAL REFERENCES

MAJOR PUBLICATION:
Roehrborn C, Oesterling J et al. The HYTRIN Community Assessment Trial study: A one-year study of terazosin versus placebo in the treatment of men with symptomatic benign prostatic hyperplasia. Urology 47:159-168, 1996.

ORIGINAL ABSTRACT: not published at AUA or EAU

OTHER IMPORTANT PUBLICATIONS:
Roehrborn C, Oesterling J et al. Serial prostate specific antigen measurements in men with concomitant benign prostatic hyperplasia during a 12 month placebo-controlled study with terazosin. Urology 50(4):556-561, 1997.

Lowe F, Olson P, Padley R. Effects of terazosin therapy on blood pressure in men with benign prostatic hyperplasia concurrently treated with other antihypertensive medications. Urology 54(1):81-85, 1999.

STUDY FUNDING: Abbott Laboratories

IMPORTANCE OF STUDY

This study was one of the first to be carried out in a community setting.
It is important because it was the first to establish that α-blockers in general and Hytrin in particular were effective in a 'real life' setting.

STUDY DESIGN

Randomised, double-blind, placebo-controlled, multicentre study. n=2084.
15 academic regional and 141 community-based private urology clinics participated
in this trial.

Following a placebo lead-in phase of 2 weeks, patients entered a 12-month
treatment period and were randomised in a double-blind fashion to receive either
terazosin once daily (n=1053) or placebo (n=1031). Terazosin doses were initiated
at 1mg for 3 days and then 2mg for 25 days. Terazosin doses were then titrated
upwards depending on therapeutic response (≤ 35% reduction in AUA-SS from
baseline) to doses of 5 or 10mg (o.d.).

OUTCOME MEASURES:
AUA-SS (0-35 point scale), AUA-BS (0-28 point scale), BPH Impact Index, QoL
and vital signs were assessed at baseline (-2), 0, 4, 8, 17, 26, 39 and 52 weeks in all
centres. In addition, for patients attending regional centres PFR, and PVR urine
and PSA levels were measured at baseline, 8, 26, 39 and 52 weeks. Treatment
failure rate (withdrawal due to persistent or worsening symptoms or need for
surgical intervention). Side effects (spontaneous reporting).

INCLUSION CRITERIA:
≥ 55 years, AUA-SS ≥ 13 and AUA-BS ≥ 8. PFR <15ml/s, voided volume ≥ 150ml.

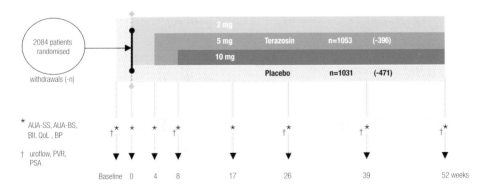

KEY RESULTS

- Statistically significant improvements were achieved in AUA-SS, AUA-BS, BII and QoL scores with terazosin treatment. AUA-SS improved by 37.8% versus 18.4% for placebo and AUA-BS by 39.6% versus 19.7%. BII improved with terazosin by 40% versus 18.9% for placebo and QoL by 33.3% versus 15.7%.

- PFR was improved by 22.9% in the terazosin group compared to 8.3% for placebo.

- Overall, 38% of terazosin patients withdrew from the trial compared to 46% of placebo patients.

- Treatment failure (lack of efficacy) occurred in 11.2% of the terazosin patients and in 25.4% of placebo treated patients (p<0.001).

- Withdrawals due to adverse events occurred in 19.7% of terazosin and 15.2% of placebo patients.

Efficacy of terazosin over 12 months in community based BPH patients with moderate to severe symptoms

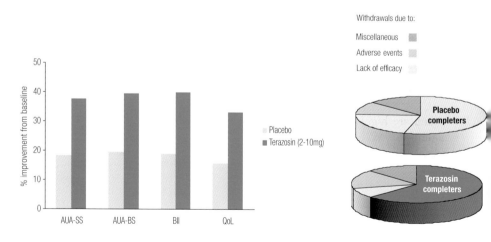

CONCLUSIONS FROM ORIGINAL REPORTS

Terazosin (2-10mg o.d.) was effective in reducing symptoms, perception of bother and impairment of QoL, in a largely community-based population of men with moderate to severe symptoms of prostatism.

The effect of terazosin was maintained over 12 months and was superior to that of placebo.

The patients from the community-based sites (urology practices) were similar to the patients from academic sites, in terms of their baseline characteristics and their response to treatment.

POPULAR CITATION: HYCAT

STRENGTHS

This was a large, well-conducted, placebo-controlled trial in a community setting. The evaluation period was much longer (1 year) than those of earlier conventional studies.

WEAKNESSES

Potentially, patients could end up at a dose of terazosin that was not producing optimal efficacy.

RELEVANCE

The data are highly representative of the likely response of BPH patients in a community or 'real life' situation, as had been suggested by studies in academic centres.

The trial that changed 5-alpha-reductase inhibitors and 'prostate shrinkage' from scientific concept to clinical reality: The utility of finasteride in the long-term management of symptomatic benign prostatic hyperplasia.

KEY TRIAL REFERENCES

MAJOR PUBLICATION:

Gormley G, Stoner E et al. The effect of finasteride in men with benign prostatic hyperplasia. N Engl J Med 327:1185-1191, 1992.

ORIGINAL ABSTRACT: not published at AUA or EAU

OTHER IMPORTANT PUBLICATIONS:

Guess H, Heyse J, Gromley G. The effect of finasteride on prostate-specific antigen in men with benign prostatic hyperplasia. Prostate 22(1):31-37, 1993.

Gormley G, Ng J et al. Effect of finasteride on prostate-specific antigen density. Urology 43(1):53-58, 1994.

Stoner E, Round E et al. Clinical experience of the detection of prostate cancer in patients with benign prostate hyperplasia treated with finasteride. The Finasteride Study Group. J Urol 151(5):1296-1300, 1994.

Stoner E. Three-year safety and efficacy data on the use of finasteride in the treatment of benign prostatic hyperplasia. Urology 43(3):284-292, 1994.

Hudson P, Boake R et al. Efficacy of finasteride is maintained in patients with benign prostatic hyperplasia treated for 5 years. The North American Finasteride Group. Urology 53(4):690-695, 1999.

STUDY FUNDING: Merck & Co

IMPORTANCE OF STUDY

This is the original clinical publication showing unequivocally the benefit of finasteride in BPH patients. The study provides clinical confirmation of the 'prostate shrinkage' approach.

STUDY DESIGN

Randomised, double-blind, placebo-controlled, multicentre study. n=895. Following a placebo lead-in phase of 2 weeks, patients were randomised to receive finasteride 5mg o.d. (n=297), finasteride 1mg o.d. (n=298) or placebo (n=300) for 12 months.

OUTCOME MEASURES:
Boyarsky (modified, 9 symptoms, scored 0-4, maximum score 36), PFR, mean flow rate, PVR urine and serum dihydrotestosterone were assessed monthly throughout the study. Prostatic volume and PSA were also assessed at baseline, 3, 6, 9 and 12 months.

INCLUSION CRITERIA:
Enlarged prostate on DRE, PFR <15ml/s, PVR urine <350ml, PSA <40μg/l.

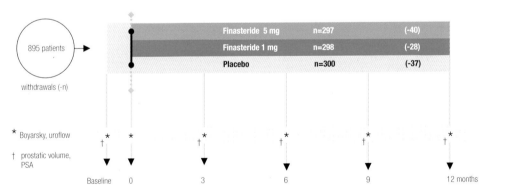

KEY RESULTS

- Finasteride 5mg resulted in significant improvements in total symptom score (↓21%), PFR (↑22%) and prostate volume (↓19%) relative to placebo after 12 months treatment.

- Finasteride 1mg resulted in significant improvement in PFR (↑23%) and prostatic volume (↓18%) versus placebo at 12 months, but not in total symptom score (↓9%).

- Patients treated with placebo experienced no change in total urinary symptom score, an 8% increase in PFR and 3% decrease in prostatic volume.

- The frequency of adverse events was similar in the 3 groups with the exception of a higher incidence of decreased libido, impotence and ejaculatory disorders in the finasteride 5mg group.

- Serum dihydrotestosterone concentrations decreased to levels present after castration soon after the initiation of finasteride therapy, the suppression being greatest in men taking the 5mg dose.

- Patients in both finasteride groups had significant reductions in median serum PSA from 3 through to 12 months (5mg group 50%, 1mg group 48%, placebo group – no change).

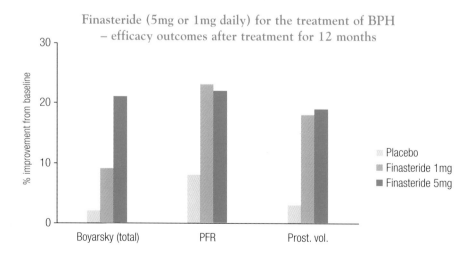

Finasteride (5mg or 1mg daily) for the treatment of BPH – efficacy outcomes after treatment for 12 months

CONCLUSIONS FROM ORIGINAL REPORTS

Finasteride therapy (5mg o.d.) resulted in significant improvements in symptoms of obstruction, in urinary flow rate and a decrease in prostatic volume.

Finasteride therapy in men with BPH resulted in sustained decreases in serum dihydrotestosterone, decreases in PSA concentrations and reduction in prostate volume.

There was a slightly increased risk of sexual dysfunction associated with the use of finasteride 5mg.

POPULAR CITATION: not applicable

STRENGTHS

A well-designed, placebo-controlled study using well characterised and validated urodynamic and symptom endpoints.

WEAKNESSES

In retrospect the study was of relatively short duration to show the optimal benefit of 'prostate shrinkage'.

Patients with atypically large prostates were enrolled.

RELEVANCE

Subsequent studies over similar periods have shown equivocal improvements in symptoms and urodynamics outcomes. However, this study is representative of the potential longer-term benefits with respect to urinary retention.

STUDY DESCRIPTOR

The first clinical trial addressing the issue of the long-term durability of drugs in the management of BPH symptomatology: Finasteride efficacy over 5 years.

KEY TRIAL REFERENCES

MAJOR PUBLICATION:
Hudson P, Boake R et al. Efficacy of finasteride is maintained in patients with benign prostatic hyperplasia treated for 5 years. The North American Finasteride Group. Urology 53(4):690-695, 1999.

ORIGINAL ABSTRACT: not published at AUA or EAU

FIRST PUBLICATION:
Gormley G, Stoner E et al. The effect of finasteride in men with benign prostatic hyperplasia. N Engl J Med 327:1185-1191, 1992.

OTHER IMPORTANT PUBLICATIONS:
McConnell J, Bruskewitz R et al. The effect of finasteride on the risk of acute urinary retention of the need for surgical treatment among men with benign prostatic hyperplasia. Finasteride Long-Term Efficacy and Safety Study Group. N Engl J Med 338(9):557-563, 1998.

Roehrborn C, McConnell J et al. Serum prostate-specific antigen concentration is a powerful predictor of acute urinary retention and need for surgery in men with clinical benign prostatic hyperplasia. PLESS Study Group. Urology 53(3):473-480, 1999.

STUDY FUNDING: Merck & Co

IMPORTANCE OF STUDY

Issues have been raised about the potential short-term (1 year) clinical benefit of finasteride and/or 'prostate shrinkage'. This study showed that there was undoubtedly a long-term benefit of this drug. These data have great significance in terms of the impact of BPH therapy on healthcare costs.

STUDY DESIGN

Open-label, long-term, multicentre extension study. n=259.
Patients (n=297) initially randomised to finasteride 5mg in a 12-month, double-blind, placebo-controlled study (see Key Clinical Trial number 4) entered this open-label extension (5mg o.d.) for an additional 4 years.

OUTCOME MEASURES:
Prostate volume was determined at baseline and annually. PFR and quasi-AUA symptom score (developed by Merck from the Merck Phase III symptom questionnaire, which was a modification of the Boyarsky scale) were assessed 6 monthly. Adverse events (including occurrence of AUR and surgery).

INCLUSION CRITERIA:
Enlarged prostate on DRE, PFR <15ml/s, PVR urine <350ml, PSA <40µg/l.

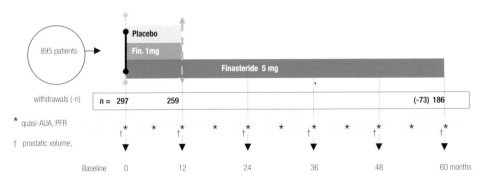

KEY RESULTS

Once daily treatment with finasteride 5mg resulted in:

- Median reduction in prostate volume being 22.7% at 12 months reaching nadir at 24 months (24.6%). This reduction was maintained through to 60 months (20.2%), compared to baseline [p<0.001].

- Symptom scores (quasi-AUA) being improved from baseline (mean 13.5) by 3.2 points at 12 months and continuing to improve until 18 months. This improvement was sustained at 60 months (4.3 points, 32%) [p<0.001].

- PFR being improved from baseline (mean 11.8ml/s) by an average of 1.6ml/s at 12 months [p<0.001]. Similarly, improvements were seen up to 18 months and sustained through to 60 months (2.3ml/s, 19%) [p<0.001]. At 60 months, 40% of patients had ≥3ml/s improvement in PFR.

- Finasteride was well tolerated. The most common AEs were related to sexual function (ejaculatory disorder, impotence, decreased libido) with a prevalence of 15.5% at 12 months (versus 8.3% for placebo), however there was no significant increase in the prevalence of sexual adverse events over time (10.1% at 60 months).

- Patients in this trial experienced a low rate of AUR (0.3-1%/year) compared to those in other long-term, placebo-controlled trials or watchful waiting.

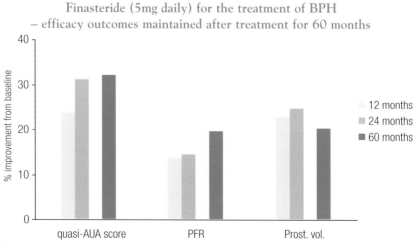

Finasteride (5mg daily) for the treatment of BPH – efficacy outcomes maintained after treatment for 60 months

CONCLUSIONS FROM ORIGINAL REPORTS

Long-term finasteride therapy (5mg o.d.) resulted in decrease in prostate volume and improved symptom scores and PFR.
Although BPH is a progressive disease, patients treated with finasteride maintained their initial improvements in these efficacy measures over 5 years.

POPULAR CITATION: not applicable

STRENGTHS

Long-term (5 years) evaluation of drug action on the symptoms of BPH.

WEAKNESSES

Like most long-term studies relatively few patients reached longer time point data read-out.

RELEVANCE

This is a highly relevant study in the determination of impact of finasteride on healthcare economics. Similar evaluations are being completed for α-blockers.

STUDY DESCRIPTOR

A key trial showing that medical management produces additional benefits to acute relief of symptoms: Finasteride: impact on acute urinary retention and surgical intervention over 4 years.

KEY TRIAL REFERENCES

MAJOR PUBLICATION:
McConnell J, Bruskewitz R et al. The effect of finasteride on the risk of acute urinary retention and the need for surgical treatment among men with benign prostatic hyperplasia. Finasteride Long-Term Efficacy and Safety Study Group. N Engl J Med 338(9):557-563, 1998.

ORIGINAL ABSTRACT: not published at AUA or EAU

FIRST PUBLICATION:
Hudson P, Boake R et al. Efficacy of finasteride is maintained in patients with benign prostatic hyperplasia treated for 5 years. The North American Finasteride Group. Urology 53(4):690-695, 1999.

OTHER IMPORTANT PUBLICATIONS:
Boyle P, Gould A, Roehrborn C. Prostate volume predicts outcome of treatment of benign prostatic hyperplasia with finasteride: meta-analysis of randomised clinical trials. Urology 46(3):398-405, 1996.

Roehrborn C, McConnell J et al. Serum prostate-specific antigen concentration is a powerful predictor of acute urinary retention and need for surgery in men with clinical benign prostatic hyperplasia. PLESS Study Group. Urology 53(3):473-480, 1999.

STUDY FUNDING: Merck & Co

IMPORTANCE OF STUDY

Earlier studies have only examined the effect of finasteride on BPH patients' symptomatology and urodynamics. This study evaluates the impact of finasteride on both urinary retention and the need for surgery. The positive effect of the drug could have an important impact on the overall healthcare costs of treating BPH patients.

STUDY DESIGN

Double-blind, randomised, placebo-controlled, long-term, multicentre study. n=3040.
In this 4-year study patients were randomised to finasteride 5mg (o.d.) or placebo, following a 1 month placebo run-in.

OUTCOME MEASURES:
PFR and quasi-AUA symptom score (developed by Merck from the Merck Phase III symptom questionnaire, which was a modification of the Boyarsky scale) and adverse events were assessed 4 monthly. Serum PSA was measured every 4 months for the first year and then 8 monthly. Prostate volume was determined annually in a subset of men. The primary endpoint was symptom score, whilst the need for surgery and the occurrence of AUR were secondary endpoints.

INCLUSION CRITERIA:
Moderate to severe symptoms of urinary obstruction, enlarged prostate on DRE, PFR <15ml/s, PSA <10ng/ml.

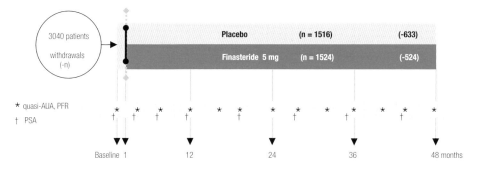

23

■ The incidence of AUR during the 4-year study period was 3% in the finasteride group and 7% in the placebo group. Thus, the risk reduction for AUR with finasteride was 57%.

■ The need for BPH surgery occurred in 5% of patients in the finasteride group during the 4-year study period compared to 10% in the placebo group (reduction in risk with finasteride 55%). The probability of undergoing transurethral prostatectomy was 49% lower in the finasteride group.

■ Symptom scores (quasi-AUA) were improved with finasteride by 3.3 points (from baseline mean, 15 points) after 4 years treatment and by 1.3 points in the placebo group [p<0.001].

■ Prostate volume was decreased in the finasteride group during the initial 12 months, with no further increase in volume up to 48 months (↓18% overall). In the placebo group, prostate volume increased continuously throughout the study (↑14% overall).

■ PFR was significantly improved in the finasteride group by an average of 1.9ml/s at 48 months versus 0.2ml/s in the placebo group [p<0.001].

■ The only drug-related AEs that occurred in 1% or more of men and that differed significantly between groups were: symptoms of sexual dysfunction, breast enlargement/tenderness and rashes. The overall incidence of prostate cancer was 5% in each group.

Reduction in risk of AUR and need for BPH surgery over 4 years
finasteride (5mg daily) *versus* placebo

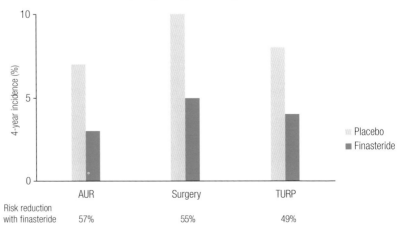

CONCLUSIONS FROM ORIGINAL REPORTS

Finasteride reduced the 4-year risk of AUR and the need for BPH surgery in men with symptoms of urinary obstruction and prostatic enlargement.
Finasteride was also effective in giving sustained improvements in symptoms and urinary flow rate and reduction in prostate volume.

POPULAR CITATION: not applicable

STRENGTHS

This study evaluates not only the acute effects of the drug on BPH symptomatology but also the clinical sequelae (urinary retention and need for surgery).
Relatively large numbers of patients reached the later time points (65%).

WEAKNESSES

Patients with relatively large prostates were included.
Interpretation of the data is dependent on relatively small absolute change in the incidence of urinary retention that is amplified by a calculation of % change.

RELEVANCE

This study is useful in calculating the benefit of long-term drug therapy on the economic cost of treating BPH patients. Similar studies are required for α-blockers.

STUDY DESCRIPTOR

Key study showing the potential of complete androgen depletion on BPH symptomatology: Leuprolide in the treatment of benign prostatic hyperplasia.

KEY TRIAL REFERENCES

MAJOR PUBLICATION:

Eri L, Tveter K. A prospective, placebo-controlled study of luteinising hormone-releasing hormone for patients with benign prostatic hyperplasia. J Urol 150:359-364, 1993.

ORIGINAL ABSTRACT: not published at AUA or EAU

OTHER IMPORTANT PUBLICATIONS

Peters C, Walsh P. The effect of nafarelin acetate, a luteinising-hormone-releasing hormone agonist on benign prostatic hyperplasia. N Engl J Med 317(10):599-604, 1987.

Eri L, Tveter K. Safety, side effects and patient acceptance of the luteinising hormone-releasing hormone agonist leuprolide in treatment of benign prostatic hyperplasia. J Urol 152(2 Pt 1):448-452, 1994.

Eri L, Urdal P, Bechensteen A. Effects of luteinising hormone releasing agonist leuprolide on lipoproteins, fibrinogen and plasminogen activator inhibitor in patients with benign prostatic hyperplasia. J Urol 154(1):100-104, 1995.

Svindland A, Eri L, Tveter K. Morphometry of benign prostatic hyperplasia during androgen suppressive therapy. Relationships among epithelial content, PSA density and clinical outcome. Scand J Nephrol Suppl 179:113-117, 1996

STUDY FUNDING: Abbott Laboratories

IMPORTANCE OF STUDY

Theoretically this study shows the maximum effect that could be achievable with androgen suppression in BPH patients. This should be equivalent to the maximal clinical benefit of a combined inhibitor of 5-α-reductase 1 and 2. The data show that androgen suppression produces good (α-blocker-like) clinical improvement by the production of near castrate DHT levels, though this is poorly tolerated by patients. Overall, this study shows that LH-RH agonists will not have an acceptable therapeutic ratio for the treatment of BPH.

STUDY DESIGN

Double-blind, placebo-controlled, randomised, equivalence study. n=55.
Following baseline evaluations patients were randomised to either leuprolide
(3.75mg depot injection) or placebo (injection) every 28 days for 24 weeks,
followed by a 24-week follow-up.

OUTCOME MEASURES:
Prostate volume and uroflow were assessed at baseline, 8, 16, 24, 36 and 48 weeks.
Symptoms scores (Madsen & Iversen, obstructive score 0-18, irritative score 0-9),
detrusor pressure and micturition patterns were assessed at baseline, 24 and 48
weeks. Hormone levels were measured at baseline, 4, 8, 12, 24, 36 and 48 weeks.

INCLUSION CRITERIA:
Moderate to severe symptoms, visual obstruction on endoscopy, prostate volume
>30ml, PFR <12ml/s, PVR urine <300ml, max. intravesicular pressure >70cm
water.

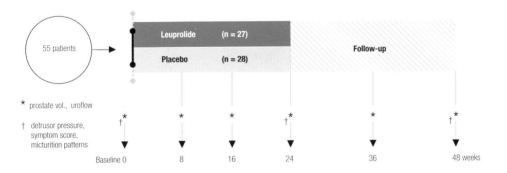

27

KEY RESULTS

- Prostate volume was decreased from baseline by 34.5% at 24 weeks with leuprolide compared to 2.6% in the placebo group. At 48 weeks, reduction in prostate volume was 16.8% with leuprolide compared to 3.1% with placebo.

- Improvements in PFR from baseline were significant throughout the study with leuprolide (23-60%) and reached significance at 24 weeks in the placebo group (25%). Increase in PFR was 32% greater than that in the placebo group at 24 weeks.

- All parameters of detrusor voiding pressure showed considerable decrease at 24 weeks for leuprolide patients and were accompanied by a 25% increase in flow rate. Most of this improvement was maintained through to 48 weeks. There was no change in pressure flow parameters in the placebo group.

- Symptom scores were improved significantly from baseline for both groups throughout the study and there was no difference between the groups at 24 weeks. Improvements in irritative symptoms for leuprolide patients reached statistical significance at 48 weeks (between group comparison).

- Notable AEs with leuprolide were hot flushes (92%, versus 4% in placebo group) and decrease or loss of erectile function (95%, versus 8% in placebo group). Erectile dysfunction was reversible in all but 2 patients of the leuprolide group. Leuprolide treatment was well tolerated despite side effects with only 1 patient withdrawal due to hot flushes.

- Serum levels of luteinising hormone and follicle-stimulating hormone decreased with leuprolide and testosterone stabilised at castrate levels. There were no changes in hormone levels in placebo patients.

Leuprolide (LH-RH agonist) versus placebo in the treatment of moderate to severe BPH – efficacy over 24 weeks therapy and 24 weeks follow-up

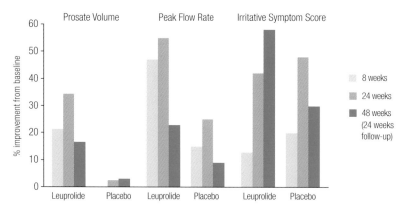

CONCLUSIONS FROM ORIGINAL REPORTS

Treatment with leuprolide was well tolerated and safe and probably the most efficient hormonal treatment for BPH available to date.
It may be recommended for BPH patients in whom surgery is contraindicated and loss of sexual function is less important.

POPULAR CITATION: not applicable

STRENGTHS

This was a well controlled, placebo study.
This drug regimen was shown to produce near castrate testosterone and dihydrotestosterone levels, indicating that an appropriate dose was used.

WEAKNESSES

Clinical evaluations were conducted over a relatively short period (48 weeks).

RELEVANCE

This study design is likely to reflect the way potentially BPH patients would be treated with LH-RH agonists. The overall clinical profile showing good efficacy but poor tolerability is likely to be predictive of larger studies. In addition, bone density must be assessed with long-term treatment.

STUDY DESCRIPTOR

Analysis of profile of one of the new generation of alpha-blockers: Alfuzosin (immediate release formulation) for the long-term medical management of benign prostatic hyperplasia.

KEY TRIAL REFERENCES

MAJOR PUBLICATION:
Jardin A, Bensadoun H et al. Long-term treatment of benign prostatic hyperplasia with alfuzosin: a 12-18 month assessment. Br J Urol 72: 615-620, 1993.

ORIGINAL ABSTRACT: not published at AUA or EAU

FIRST PUBLICATION:
Jardin A, Bensadoun H et al. Alfuzosin for treatment of benign prostatic hypertrophy. Lancet 337:1457-1461, 1991.

OTHER IMPORTANT PUBLICATION:
Jardin A, Bensadoun H et al. Long-term treatment of benign prostatic hyperplasia with a 24-30 month survey. Br J Urol 74(5):579-584, 1994.

STUDY FUNDING: Synthélabo Ltd

IMPORTANCE OF STUDY

This study unequivocally shows the benefit and durability of alfuzosin on LUTS. In addition the study shows that there is little sign of drug-induced haemodynamic effects.

STUDY DESIGN

Open-label, multicentre study. n=131.
Patients recruited from a 6-month multicentre, double-blind, placebo-controlled study (n=518). Of the 131 men entering this open study, 68 had received alfuzosin (7.5-10mg daily) and 63 placebo during the preceding controlled trial.
During this open study all patients received 2.5mg (t.i.d.), though the evening dose could be doubled depending on therapeutic response and safety. Patients who had received alfuzosin during the controlled study continued on their previous dose.

OUTCOME MEASURES:
Boyarsky scale (seven symptoms from the scale were assessed, scored 0-3, maximum score 21), BP (including occurrence of asymptomatic postural hypotension) were assessed at baseline, 3, 6, 9 and 12 months. PFR, mean flow rate, voided volume, residual urine, biochemistry (assessed at baseline, 6 and 12 months). Side effects (spontaneous reporting).

INCLUSION CRITERIA:
Diagnosis of BPH based on medical history and physical examination. Boyarsky total symptom score >6. Controlled hypertensive patients included (but not those taking α- or β-blockers).

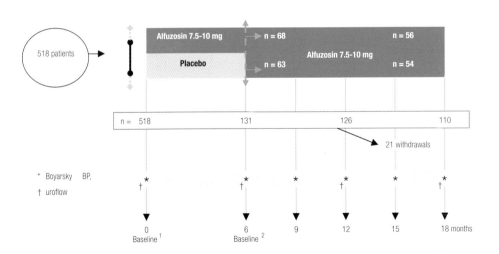

KEY RESULTS

- After 12 months treatment with alfuzosin (n=122), all obstructive and irritative symptoms according to the Boyarsky scale were significantly improved. Mean decrease in total score for this patient group was –3.68 points.

- Mean flow rate (↑ 34%, n=46) and residual urine (↓ 49%, n=35) were significantly improved after 12 months treatment. PFR in the whole population was not significantly increased, but in the more obstructed patients significant improvements (↑ 58%) were seen.

- For the 56 patients who received alfuzosin for 18 months, improvements in voiding symptoms were sustained.

- Only 5.3% of patients experienced vasodilatory side effects and none of these led to withdrawal from the study.

- No treatment-related side effects were reported during long-term treatment with alfuzosin.

Long-term efficacy of alfuzosin in patients with BPH
(7.5–10mg/day for 12 months)

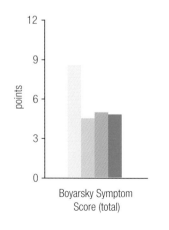

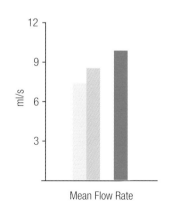

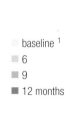

baseline [1]
6
9
12 months

CONCLUSIONS FROM ORIGINAL REPORTS

Alfuzosin has a sustained beneficial effect on voiding symptoms and appears to be safe when administered long-term in BPH patients.

POPULAR CITATION: not applicable

STRENGTHS

A well designed placebo-controlled study.

WEAKNESSES

The duration of the study was relatively short and the patient numbers were low.

RELEVANCE

This study is predictive of the clinical performance of alfuzosin in urological practice. Alfuzosin is shown to be effective and has little cardiovascular activity.

STUDY DESCRIPTOR

Important trial analysing long-term durability of response and patient compliance: Alfuzosin (immediate release formulation) for the treatment of benign prostatic hyperplasia, a long-term follow-up of patients in a community-based setting.

KEY TRIAL REFERENCES

MAJOR PUBLICATION:
Lukacs B, Grange J et al. History of 7,093 patients with lower urinary tract symptoms related to benign prostatic hyperplasia treated with alfuzosin in general practice up to 3 years. Eur Urol 37:183-190, 2000

FIRST PUBLICATION:
Lukacs B, McCarthy C et al. Long-term quality of life in patients with benign prostatic hypertrophy: preliminary results of a cohort survey of 7,093 patients treated with an alpha-blocker, alfuzosin. Eur Urol 24(suppl) 10:34-40, 1993.

OTHER IMPORTANT PUBLICATIONS:
Lukacs B, Blondin P et al. Safety profile of 3 months' therapy with alfuzosin in 13,389 patients suffering from benign prostatic hypertrophy. Eur Urol 29:29-35, 1996.

Lukacs B, Comet et al. Health related quality of life in benign prostatic hyperplasia patients treated for 2 years with alfuzosin. J Epidemiol Biostat 2:203-211, 1997.

Lukacs B, Grange J, McCarthy C. Prospective follow-up of 3,228 patients suffering from clinical benign prostatic hyperplasia (BPH) treated for 3 years with alfuzosin in general practice. Prog Urol 2:271-280, 1999.

STUDY FUNDING: Synthélabo Ltd

IMPORTANCE OF STUDY

Traditionally, BPH trials are conducted over short periods in specialist urological practices. This study shows that the efficacy of alfuzosin is maintained over a long period in a real-life situation. Most previous studies have analysed data from only relatively few patients reaching the end point but this study reports on 2579 patients who completed 36 months of treatment.

STUDY DESIGN

Open-label, multicentre, GP-based, long-term trial. n=7093.
Patients recruited at 1812 GP centres. This study analysed 4 patient populations
(A, B, C, & D), who received treatment for 3, 12, 24 and 36 months. (n= 7093,
5849, 4591 and 3228 respectively).
Patients received alfuzosin immediate-release formulation tablets 2.5mg t.i.d.
(7.5mg daily).

OUTCOME MEASURES:
Drop-out rate, reasons for drop-out and incidence of AUR and prostate surgery.
Symptoms were measured using the 9 items of the Boyarsky scale plus an additional
item (straining to void). These symptoms were scored 0-4 (maximum score 40) and
were assessed at baseline, 1, 3, 6, 12, 18, 24, 30 and 36 months. Patients were
stratified according to symptom severity; mild (0-13), moderate (14-26) and severe
(27-40). QoL questionnaire (Urolife – BPHQL20, max. score 200) assessed at
baseline, 3, 6, 12, 18, 24, 30 and 36 months. BP & HR were measured at each visit.
Side effects (spontaneous reporting).

INCLUSION CRITERIA:
Men <85 years with a clinical diagnosis of BPH. Patients taking other α-blockers
were excluded.

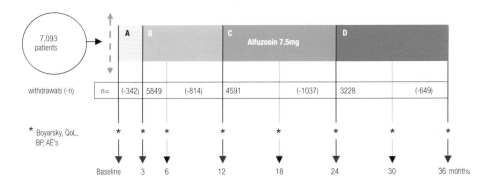

KEY RESULTS

- Over 36% of the patients (n=2579) completed 36 months of treatment. The overall drop-out rate (per month) in each of the patient populations was: A, 1.6%; B, 1.2%; C, 0.9% and D, 0.6%.

- In population D (36 months) the symptom profile improved with treatment: of 1528 patients with moderate symptoms at baseline, 84.7% were improved, 14.7% clinically stable and 0.6% worse. Of the 279 patients classified as severe at baseline, 78.1% and 21.5% reported mild and moderate symptoms respectively at 36 months.

- The class of symptom severity was not predictive for drop-outs: in patients with severe symptoms the number of patients in each of the study populations who dropped out were 3.5, 12.6, 20, and 14.3% compared to 4.2, 13.7, 22.9 and 14% for patients with moderate symptoms. Symptom severity was not predictive of progression to surgery or the occurrence of AUR.

- In population D, the main reason for withdrawal was lack of improvement in QoL as measured by magnitude of effect.

Follow-up of BPH patients treated with alfuzosin for up to 3 years, distribution of withdrawals from treatment relative to baseline symptom class (mild, moderate and severe)

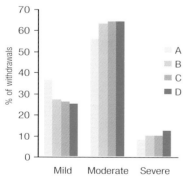

Distribution of withdrawals relative to baseline symptom classes and study population (A: 3, B:12, C:24, D:36 months)

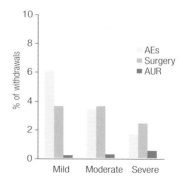

Distribution of withdrawals over 36 months due to AEs, progression to surgery and occurrence of AUR relative to baseline symptom classes

CONCLUSIONS FROM ORIGINAL REPORTS

The magnitude of reductions in symptom score and HRQL were sustained over 3 years treatment with alfuzosin.

For patients receiving long-term (36 months) treatment with alfuzosin in the community setting, the reasons for withdrawal from treatment did not correlate with symptom severity.

POPULAR CITATION: not applicable

STRENGTHS

A good long-term study conducted in a primary care setting. A relatively large number of patients completed the study (n=2579).

WEAKNESSES

There was no comparison with placebo or watchful waiting.
This study used the original (immediate-release) formulation of alfuzosin.

RELEVANCE

The setting and powering of the study is such that it is likely to be predictive of the actual clinical benefit of the α-blocker in the hands of the primary care physician. GPs account for over 85% of the prescriptions for α-blockers.

STUDY DESCRIPTOR

First study addressing the impact of alpha-blockers on the 20-30% of patients who are controlled hypertensives: Medical management of benign prostatic hyperplasia with doxazosin in normotensive and controlled hypertensive patients.

KEY TRIAL REFERENCES

MAJOR PUBLICATION:

Kaplan S, Meade-D'Alisera P et al. Doxazosin in physiologically and pharmacologically normotensive men with benign prostatic hyperplasia. Urology 46:512-517, 1995.

FIRST PUBLICATIONS:

Kaplan S, Soldo K, Olsson C. Effect of dosing regimen on efficacy and safety of doxazosin in normotensive men with symptomatic prostatism: a pilot study. Urology 44(3): 348-352, 1994.

Kaplan S, Soldo K, Olsson C. Terazosin and doxazosin in normotensive men with symptomatic prostatism: a pilot study to determine the effect of dosing regimen on efficacy and safety. Eur Urol 28(3):223-228, 1995.

OTHER IMPORTANT PUBLICATIONS:

Lepor H, Kaplan S et al. Doxazosin for benign prostatic hyperplasia: Long term efficacy and safety in normotensive and hypertensive patients. J Urol 157:525-530, 1997.

Kaplan S, Meade-D'Alisera P. Tolerability of alpha-blockade with doxazosin as a therapeutic option for symptomatic benign prostatic hyperplasia in the elderly patient: a pooled analysis of seven double-blind, placebo-controlled studies. J Gerontol A Biol Sci Med Sci 53(3):M201-206, 1998.

STUDY FUNDING: Pfizer Ltd

IMPORTANCE OF STUDY

A question often raised by physicians is the impact of an α-blocker on the blood pressure control of BPH patients receiving other antihypertensive medication. This study shows that doxazosin produces no clinically further reductions in blood pressure in these circumstances.

STUDY DESIGN

Pooled results of 2 open-label, parallel, randomised studies. n=63 (31 normotensive, 32 controlled hypertensives). Pharmacologically normotensive patients (controlled hypertensives) were taking a single antihypertensive agent (Ca channel blockers, ACE inhibitors or β-blockers).

Study 1: Patients randomised to AM or PM dosing. 3-week titration period followed by 3 months treatment with doxazosin (4mg o.d.). Extension period, 12 months.

Study 2: Patients randomised to AM or PM dosing and to 4mg or 8mg (o.d.) dosing groups. 3-4 week dose titration followed by 3 months treatment. Extension period, 12 months.

OUTCOME MEASURES:
Blood pressure, PFR, Boyarsky symptom score (9 symptoms, scored 0-3, maximum score 27), measured at baseline, 1 month and 3 months and then 3 monthly.

INCLUSION CRITERIA:
50-80 years, BPH diagnosis, Boyarsky score < 8, PFR 5-15ml/s, voided volume ≥ 150ml, DBP <90mmHg.

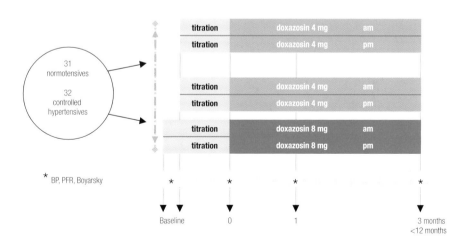

KEY RESULTS

■ The small reductions in systolic and diastolic blood pressures at 1 month and 3 months were recorded in both physiologically and pharmacologically normotensive patients. For physiologically normotensive patients mean reductions in blood pressures at 1 and 3 months were –4.9/–4.7mmHg and –4.0/–2.9mmHg and for pharmacologically normotensive patients –2.3/–2.7mmHg and –2.1/–2.4mmHg respectively.

■ These changes from baseline were statistically significant but clinically unimportant and there was no difference between groups. There was no tendency for the effects to increase between 1 and 3 months.

■ Clinically and statistically significant improvements occurred in PFR and Boyarsky symptom score by 1 month and further improvements were seen after 3 months. Improvements in these efficacy measures were not affected by time of dosing (AM or PM).

Changes in systolic and diastolic blood pressure in pharmacologically and physiologically normotensive men with BPH following 1 month and 3 months treatment with doxazosin

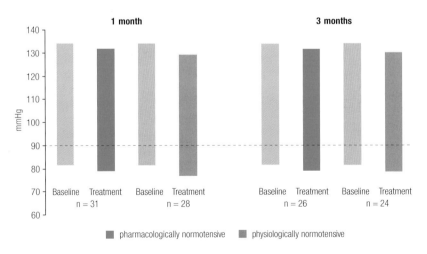

CONCLUSIONS FROM ORIGINAL REPORTS

Doxazosin may be used to treat BPH in men who are either physiologically normotensive or whose hypertension is controlled by other antihypertensive medications, without further clinical reduction in blood pressure.

Evening dosing with doxazosin does not diminish efficacy and may enhance tolerability.

POPULAR CITATION: not applicable

STRENGTHS

These are well-controlled clinical trials in specialist (urological) settings.

WEAKNESSES

These studies were open label and the actions of doxazosin were only studied in combination with antihypertensive monotherapies.

RELEVANCE

This study is particularly relevant to the management of BPH patients with co-morbid hypertension in the primary care setting. The data presented here show that doxazosin can be safely added to existing antihypertensive medication without producing an additive effect on blood pressure control.

STUDY DESCRIPTOR

Trial analysing the impact of alpha-blockers on blood pressure control in the 40% of patients who may be controlled or uncontrolled hypertensives: Medical management of benign prostatic hyperplasia with doxazosin, in normotensive patients and in patients with concomitant hypertension.

KEY TRIAL REFERENCES

MAJOR PUBLICATION:
Kirby RS. Doxazosin in benign prostatic hyperplasia: effects on blood pressure and urinary flow in normotensive and hypertensive men. Urology 46: 182-186, 1995

ORIGINAL ABSTRACT:
Kirby RS, Chapple C, Christmas T. Doxazosin: minimal blood pressure effects in normotensive BPH patients. J Urol 149 (suppl. 886): 434A, 1993.

FIRST PUBLICATION:
Chapple C, Carter P, Christmas T et al. A three month double-blind study of doxazosin as treatment for benign prostatic bladder outlet obstruction. Br J Urol 75(6):809-810, 1995.

OTHER IMPORTANT PUBLICATIONS:
Janknegt R, Chapple C. Efficacy and safety of the alpha-1 blocker doxazosin in the treatment of benign prostatic hyperplasia. Analysis of 5 studies. Doxazosin Study Groups. Eur Urol 24(3):319-326, 1993.

Gillenwater J, Conn R et al. Doxazosin for the treatment of benign prostatic hyperplasia in patients with mild to moderate essential hypertension: a double-blind, placebo-controlled, dose response multicentre study. J Urol 154(1):110-115, 1995.

STUDY FUNDING: Pfizer Ltd

IMPORTANCE OF STUDY

A key issue often raised by primary care physicians is the impact of α-blockers on blood pressure. This study shows that in the 40% of BPH patients who have concomitant hypertension, doxazosin produces a beneficial blood pressure lowering effect. Importantly, this study also shows that doxazosin has little impact on the blood pressure in normotensive patients.

STUDY DESIGN

Pooled results of 2 double-blind, placebo-controlled studies. n=232 (doxazosin: 22 hypertensive, 92 normotensive and placebo: 29 hypertensive, 81 normotensive). Following a washout period of at least 1 week patients were randomised to doxazosin (titrated up to 4mg/day) or placebo for 9-12 weeks treatment.

OUTCOME MEASURES:
Blood pressure, mean and maximum flow rates measured at baseline, 2, 4, 8 and 12 weeks.

INCLUSION CRITERIA:
50-80 years, enlarged prostate on physical examination, nocturia (≥2), frequency of micturition (≥10/24hrs), PFR <15ml/s. Hypertensive patients DBP> 90mmHg, normotensive DBP <90mmHg.

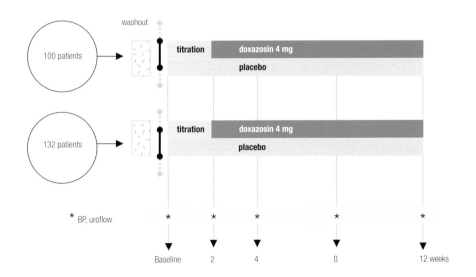

KEY RESULTS

- Doxazosin produced a clinically significant reduction in blood pressure only in the hypertensive patients. Mean reduction (from baseline to endpoint) in blood pressures (sitting) were: for hypertensive patients –19/–10 mmHg and for normotensive patients –5/–4 mmHg (similar to normotensive placebo group).

- Doxazosin had similar effects on uroflow in both hypertensive and normotensive patients. Maximum flow rate increased by 23% in hypertensive patients and by 28% in normotensive patients treated with doxazosin. Mean flow rate increased by 22% and 29% respectively in hypertensive and normotensive patients.

Changes in systolic and diastolic blood pressures in hypertensive and normotensive men with BPH following treatment with doxazosin or placebo

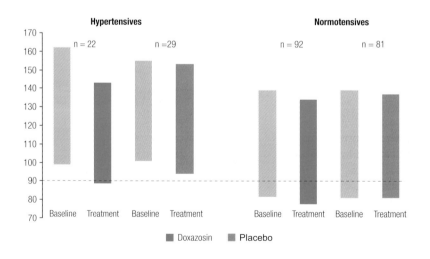

CONCLUSIONS FROM ORIGINAL REPORTS

Doxazosin is effective in reducing symptoms of BPH in both normotensive and hypertensive men, irrespective of blood pressure.

Doxazosin produces clinically and statistically significant reduction in blood pressure in hypertensive men but clinically insignificant reduction in normotensive men.

POPULAR CITATION: not applicable

STRENGTHS

This study represents a rigorous evaluation of the effect of doxazosin on blood pressure in a carefully controlled clinical setting.

WEAKNESSES

The hypertensive cohort was only 51 patients out of a total 232 men, of which only 22 were randomised to doxazosin.

Although blood pressure was measured on several occasions this was only at a single time point.

RELEVANCE

This study is representative of the co-morbidity between BPH and hypertension, likely to be seen by both urologists and primary care physicians.

Additionally, this study shows that doxazosin has negligible effects on blood pressure in normotensive patients. This has subsequently been confirmed in longer-term studies.

STUDY DESCRIPTOR

The definitive clinical trial examining the durability of the BPH symptom improvement and hypertensive control produced by alpha-blockers: Long-term medical management of benign prostatic hyperplasia with doxazosin in hypertensive and normotensive patients.

KEY TRIAL REFERENCES

MAJOR PUBLICATION:
Lepor H, Kaplan S et al. Doxazosin for benign prostatic hyperplasia: Long-term efficacy and safety in normotensive and hypertensive patients. J Urol 157:525-530, 1997.

FIRST PUBLICATIONS:
Kaplan S, Meade-D'Alisera P et al. Doxazosin in physiologically and pharmacologically normotensive men with benign prostatic hyperplasia. Urology 46:512-517, 1995.

Gillenwater J, Conn R et al. Doxazosin for the treatment of prostatic hyperplasia in patients with mild to moderate essential hypertension: a double-blind, placebo-controlled, dose-response multicentre study. J Urol 154:129-130, 1995.

OTHER IMPORTANT PUBLICATIONS:
Mobley D, Kaplan S et al. Effect of doxazosin on the symptoms of benign hyperplasia: results from three double-blind, placebo-controlled studies. Int J Clin Pract 51:282-288, 1997.

Fawzy A, Vashi et al. Clinical correlation of maximal urinary flow rate and plasma doxazosin concentrations in the treatment of benign prostatic hyperplasia. Multicentre Study Group. Urology 53:329-335, 1999.

STUDY FUNDING: Pfizer Ltd

IMPORTANCE OF STUDY

Earlier studies showed that doxazosin produces a rapid and effective relief of the lower urinary tract symptoms (LUTS) associated with BPH. This study shows that the benefit is durable and efficacy is maintained for at least 4 years.

STUDY DESIGN

Open-labelled, multicentre extension study. n=450 (178 hypertensive, 272 normotensive).

Patients recruited from 3 multicentre, double-blind, placebo-controlled studies.

Patients entered this extension study 1-2 weeks after completion of one of the 3 double-blind studies, no study medication was administered during this washout phase. Doxazosin was initiated at 1mg and titrated at 2 weekly intervals up to a maximum of 8mg (o.d.) for normotensives and 12mg (o.d.) for hypertensives. After dose stabilisation patients entered the stable dose efficacy phase (duration 3-48 months). Median treatment periods were 26.5 months for hypertensives and 22 months for normotensives. Mean doses at endpoint were 6.4mg and 4mg daily for hypertensive and normotensive patients respectively.

OUTCOME MEASURES:

Blood pressure, heart rate, mean and maximum flow rates, voided volume, post-void residual volume, symptom severity and bothersomeness (AUA-based or a modified Boyarsky-based questionnaire) and safety were assessed at baseline, 1, 3, 6, 9, 12 months and 6-monthly up to a maximum of 48 months.

INCLUSION CRITERIA:

>45 years. Hypertensive patients: PFR 5-15ml/s, voided volume 150-500ml, micturition frequency >4/daytime, nocturia >2, DBP 90-114mmHg. Normotensive patients: PFR 5-15ml/s, voided volume 125-500ml, PVR <250ml, DBP <90mmHg.

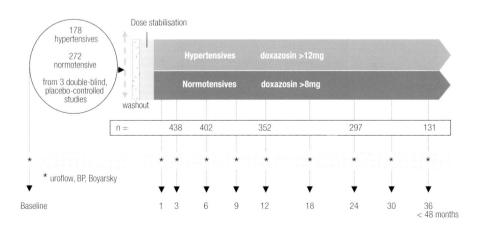

KEY RESULTS

- Doxazosin treatment resulted in significant improvements (baseline to endpoint) in mean and maximum flow rates (1.0ml and 1.9ml/s respectively, all patients), which were sustained at 45-48 months. Reductions in post-void residual urine (–27.7ml, all patients) were also seen at efficacy endpoint.

- Statistically significant and sustained improvements in symptom scores were achieved with doxazosin (bothersomeness, 14.8% overall group endpoint, 13.2% for those patients who had completed 45-48 months treatment).

- Clinically and statistically significant reduction in blood pressure was sustained in hypertensive patients (8/11mmHg, standing). Blood pressure reductions in normotensive patients (4/2mmHg, standing) were not clinically significant.

- Compared to the preceding double-blind, placebo-controlled studies, the overall incidence of adverse events did not increase with increasing duration of treatment. Fewer normotensive patients than hypertensive withdrew from this study due to adverse events, 15.1% versus 19.1% respectively. Almost 90% of all adverse events were assessed by the investigators to be mild/moderate in severity.

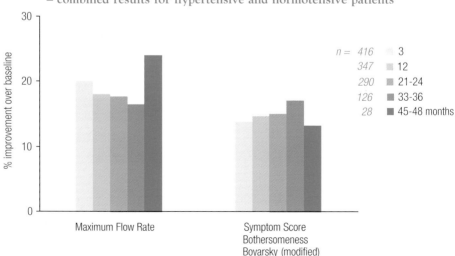

Long-term efficacy of doxazosin in the treatment of BPH – combined results for hypertensive and normotensive patients

$n =$	
416	3
347	12
290	21-24
126	33-36
28	45-48 months

CONCLUSIONS FROM ORIGINAL REPORTS

Doxazosin was significantly effective and well tolerated in the long-term treatment (up to 48 months) of BPH, for both normotensive and hypertensive men.

POPULAR CITATION: not applicable

STRENGTHS

Conventionally efficacy is measured over 12 weeks. This study evaluates efficacy over periods up to and including 48 months.

WEAKNESSES

As in the case of all long-term studies, relatively few patients have been on therapy for the full 4 years (n = 28 at 45-48 months).
This study was also open-label, physician and patient being aware of the potential effects of the medication.

RELEVANCE

A perceived disadvantage of α-blocker therapy is that any benefit could be transient and only maintained for a few months. This study shows that in a situation likely to be representative of primary care, the effect of doxazosin is maintained over much longer periods. This could be important in the development of arguments relating to healthcare economics.

STUDY DESCRIPTOR

First clinical trial showing the impact of novel formulation (i.e. pharmacokinetic manipulation) on therapeutic response: Alfuzosin (prolonged release formulation) in the treatment of benign prostatic hyperplasia.

KEY TRIAL REFERENCES

MAJOR PUBLICATION:

van Kerrebroeck P, Jardin A et al. Efficacy and safety of new prolonged release formulation of alfuzosin 10mg once daily versus alfuzosin 2.5mg thrice daily and placebo in patients with symptomatic benign prostatic hyperplasia. Eur Urol 37:306-313, 2000.

ORIGINAL ABSTRACT:

van Kerrebroeck P. Efficacy and tolerability of a new once-a-day formulation of alfuzosin for LUTS suggestive of BPH. AUA Abstracts: 973, 2000.

SUBSEQUENT ABSTRACT:

van Kerrebroeck P, Jardin A et al. 12-month study of efficacy and safety of a new once-a-day formulation of alfuzosin for symptomatic BPH. AUA Abstracts: 970, 2000.

OTHER IMPORTANT PUBLICATION:

van Kerrebroeck P. The efficacy and safety of a new once-a-day formulation of an alpha-blocker. Eur Urol 39 (suppl. 6):19-26, 2001.

STUDY FUNDING: Synthélabo Ltd

IMPORTANCE OF STUDY

This is a key comparator study showing the impact of drug formulation (immediate release versus prolonged release) on the clinical profile of an α-blocker, alfuzosin. This study provides important data for physicians, enabling them to make an informed decision on 'switching' to the new formulation of alfuzosin.

STUDY DESIGN

Randomised, double-blind, placebo-controlled, multicentre, multinational study. n=447.
Patients recruited at 48 urology centres in 4 European countries. Following a 1-month, placebo-controlled run-in patients were randomised to alfuzosin 10mg o.d. (n=143), alfuzosin 2.5mg t.i.d. (n=150) or placebo (n=154) for 3 months treatment. 63% of patients were receiving at least one concomitant medication and 30% were receiving antihypertensive medication.

OUTCOME MEASURES:
IPSS (maximum score 35), QoL index, uroflow and PVR and BP were assessed at baseline, 2, 4, 8 and 12 weeks. Side effects (spontaneous reporting).

INCLUSION CRITERIA:
>50 years, IPSS ≥ 13, PFR 5-12ml/s, PVR ≤ 350ml. Controlled hypertensive patients included. Patients taking concomitant medications included (but not those taking α-blockers, androgen, antiandrogens, 5α-reductase inhibitors, LH-RH analogues).

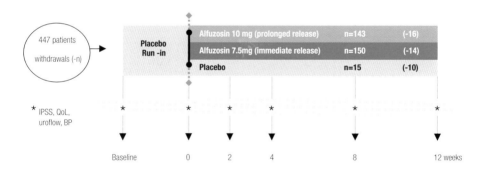

KEY RESULTS

- Both formulations of alfuzosin significantly improved symptoms versus placebo as assessed by IPSS. Improvements over baseline scores after 3 months treatment were: prolonged release 40%, immediate release 38%, placebo 28%.

- Alfuzosin treatment was efficacious on both IPSS voiding and filling symptom subscores.

- Global QoL scores were also improved: 33%, 30% and 18% for prolonged release, immediate release and placebo respectively.

- PFR was also significantly improved with alfuzosin treatment compared to placebo: prolonged release 24.5%, immediate release 36%, placebo 15%.

- Both formulations of alfuzosin were well tolerated and the incidence of vasodilatory side effects was less with the prolonged release formulation (prolonged release 6.3%, immediate release 9.4%, placebo 2.6%).

Alfuzosin, prolonged release, once daily formulation (PR) – efficacy and safety over 3 months treatment, compared to immediate release, thrice daily formulation (IR) and placebo

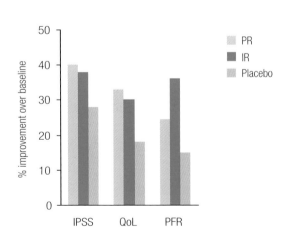

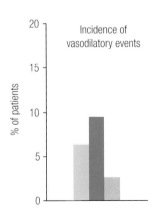

CONCLUSIONS FROM ORIGINAL REPORTS

The prolonged release formulation of alfuzosin (10mg o.d.) has a beneficial effect on LUTS associated with BPH and is as effective as the immediate release formulation (2.5mg t.i.d.).

It has an improved cardiovascular profile compared to the immediate release formulation and did not require dose titration.

This improved safety profile allows the same dose to be used in all patients and provides patients with the convenience of once daily administration.

POPULAR CITATION: not applicable

STRENGTHS

This is one of only a few side-by-side comparator studies, comparing two formulations of the same drug and placebo.

WEAKNESSES

Only one dose of each formulation was used.

RELEVANCE

An elegant study offering the decision-maker the key comparative data on the existing (immediate release) and new (prolonged release) formulations of alfuzosin. In particular, this study shows the reduced cardiovascular side effects of the new formulation that may offer an advantage to patient and physician.

STUDY DESCRIPTOR

Definitive clinical trial comparing the effects of standard and sustained release formulations on BPH symptom improvement: Doxazosin (controlled release formulation) for the treatment of benign prostatic hyperplasia.

KEY TRIAL REFERENCES

MAJOR PUBLICATION:
Kirby RS, Andersen M. A combined analysis of double-blind trials of the efficacy and tolerability of doxazosin-gastrointestinal therapeutic system, doxazosin standard and placebo in patients with benign prostatic hyperplasia. Br J Urol 87:192-200, 2001.

ORIGINAL ABSTRACT:
Gratzke P. Doxazosin gastrointestinal therapeutic system (GITS) in benign prostatic hyperplasia (BPH). AUA Abstracts:1395, 1999.

FIRST PUBLICATION:
Andersen M, Dahlstrand C, Hoye K. Double-blind trial of the efficacy and tolerability of doxazosin in the gastrointestinal therapeutic system, doxazosin standard and placebo in patients with benign prostatic hyperplasia. Eur Urol 38:400-409, 2000.

Gratzke P, Kirby R et al. Doxazosin (GITS) versus regular doxazosin standard in benign prostatic hyperplasia: restoring urine flow and sexual function. Munchener Medizinische Wochenschrift 2000, in press.

OTHER IMPORTANT PUBLICATIONS:
Os I, Stokke H. Effects of doxazosin in the gastrointestinal therapeutic system formulations versus doxazosin standard and placebo in mild-to-moderate hypertension. J Cardiovasc Pharmacol 33:791-797, 1999.

Os I, Stokke H. Doxazosin GITS compared with doxazosin standard and placebo in patients with mild hypertension. Blood Press 8(3):184-191, 1999.

STUDY FUNDING: Pfizer Inc

IMPORTANCE OF STUDY

Although a composite of 2 clinical trials, this study makes an important contribution to our understanding of modern drug development. Data show that novel formulations can substantially impact the clinical profile (therapeutic ratio) of α-blockers (in this case doxazosin).

STUDY DESIGN

Integrated analysis of results of 2 parallel, double-blind, multicentre studies. n=1475.
Both studies involved a 2-week placebo washout, a 2-week single-blind placebo run-in followed by 13 weeks of double-blind treatment. One study (n=795) compared doxazosin GITS, doxazosin standard and placebo. The other study (n=680) compared doxazosin GITS and doxazosin standard. In both studies doxazosin GITS was initiated at 4mg o.d. and increased to 8mg o.d. after 7 weeks if required, to attain optimal response. Doxazosin standard was initiated at 1mg o.d. and titrated to 4mg o.d. at 3 weeks and to 8mg o.d. at week 7 as required, to achieve optimal symptom control.

OUTCOME MEASURES:
In all patients, IPSS (maximum score 35) plus one IPSS QoL question (score 0-6) and PFR were assessed at baseline, weeks 3, 7 and 13. A physician-rated impression of global efficacy (score 1-4) was performed at baseline and end of study. Tolerability (BP, ECG, haematology, biochemistry) and AEs were monitored throughout the studies. IIEF was assessed at baseline and 13 weeks in the GITS vs standard study.

INCLUSION CRITERIA:
50-80 years, PFR ≥5 ml/s and ≤15ml/s, IPSS ≥ 12. Enlarged prostate on DRE for the GITS vs standard study.

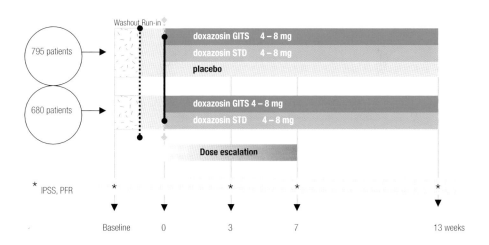

KEY RESULTS

- Both formulations of doxazosin significantly improved symptoms of BPH as determined by IPSS, with 45% reduction in scores from baseline to final visit, compared to 34% reduction with placebo.

- The GITS formulation gave significantly greater improvements in IPSS during the first 3 weeks than the standard formulation, and comparable symptom reductions at 7 weeks and thereafter.

- Both formulations of doxazosin resulted in similar improvements in PFR at final visit that were significantly greater than placebo (approx. GITS 27%, standard 25% and placebo 11%).

- Doxazosin GITS appeared to produce maximal effects on flow rates earlier (by week 3) than standard formulation and to a degree that was comparable with that achieved with the standard formulation at final visit.

- Overall improvement of efficacy (physician assessed) from baseline to final visit was considered to be excellent or good in 61.2% of GITS patients, 61.9% for standard formulation and 37.5% for placebo, for intention to treat analysis.

- For those patients reporting a sexual dysfunction at baseline (GITS vs standard study) there were significant improvements in sexual function with both formulations of doxazosin.

- The incidence of AEs in patients treated with the GITS formulation (41.4%) was similar to that of placebo (39.1%) and lower than that of the standard formulation (53.6%). Treatment-related AEs occurred in fewer GITS patients than those taking the standard formulation (GITS 16.1%, standard 25.3% and placebo 7.7%).

Doxazosin GITS compared to doxazosin standard formulation and placebo
– efficacy outcomes over 13 weeks

GITS formulation gives earlier improvements than standard formulation

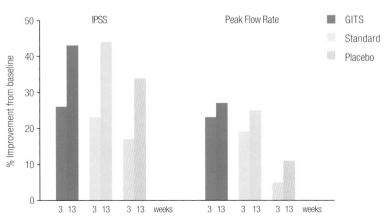

CONCLUSIONS FROM ORIGINAL REPORTS

The GITS formulation of doxazosin was significantly more effective than placebo and as effective as the standard formulation in improving symptoms of BPH and PFR.

Both formulations of doxazosin improved sexual function in patients with sexual dysfunction at baseline.

Doxazosin GITS had a therapeutic effect equivalent to that of the standard formulation but with fewer titration steps and a slightly lower incidence of adverse events.

POPULAR CITATION: not applicable

STRENGTHS

Two excellent studies involving the drug under examination (GITS formulation), a comparator agent (standard formulation) and placebo.

WEAKNESSES

Complete dose ranges were not employed, therefore direct quantification of efficacy is not possible.

RELEVANCE

This study design is representative of a dosing regimen likely to be used in the management of BPH patients and their co-morbidities. Parameters measured are those that impact on patients' perception of efficacy and tolerability and are therefore likely to reflect overall compliance.

STUDY DESCRIPTOR

First and definitive study examining the potential benefits of a combination of alpha-blockade and 5-alpha-reductase inhibition: Comparison of terazosin, finasteride and both in combination, for the treatment of benign prostatic hyperplasia.

KEY TRIAL REFERENCES

MAJOR PUBLICATION:
Lepor H, Williford W et al. The efficacy of terazosin, finasteride or both in benign prostatic hyperplasia. N Engl J Med 335:533-539, 1996.

OTHER IMPORTANT PUBLICATIONS:
Lepor H, Williford W et al. The impact of medical therapy on bother, quality of life and global outcome, and factors predicting response. Veterans Affairs Cooperative Studies Benign Prostatic Hyperplasia Study Group. J Urol 160(4):1358-1367, 1998.

Debruyne F, Jardin A et al. Sustained-release alfuzosin, finasteride and the combination of both in the treatment of benign prostatic hyperplasia. European ALFIN Study Group. Eur Urol 34(3):169-175, 1998.

Brawer M, Lin D et al. Effect of finasteride on serum PSA: results of VA cooperative study #359. Prostate 39(4):234-239, 1999.

Lepor H, Jones K, Williford W. The mechanism of adverse events associated with terazosin: an analysis of the Veterans Affairs Cooperative Study. J Urol 163(4):1134-1137, 2000.

STUDY FUNDING: Merck & Co, Abbott Laboratories, Veterans Affairs Medical Research Service

IMPORTANCE OF STUDY

This is the definitive combination study showing the clinical effect of a combination of α-blocker and 5-α-reductase inhibitor. The results showed that there is little advantage of adding the two drugs (finasteride and terazosin) beyond that of terazosin alone. Certainly there would be an obvious cost disadvantage of such a combination that would not be justified by the clinical benefit.

STUDY DESIGN

Randomised, double-blind, placebo-controlled, multicentre study. n=1229.
Following a single-blind, placebo lead-in phase of 4 weeks, patients were randomised in a double-blind fashion to terazosin 10mg o.d. (n=305), finasteride 5mg o.d. (n=310), terazosin/finasteride combination (n=309) or placebo (n=305) for 12 months treatment. Terazosin doses were titrated up to 10mg during the initial 2 weeks of the treatment period and dose reduction was permitted for terazosin or finasteride in the event of adverse events.

OUTCOME MEASURES:
AUA-SS (7 symptoms, 35 maximum score), uroflow, PVR urine, AEs, compliance and vital signs were assessed at baseline, 2, 4, 13, 26, 39 and 52 weeks. AEs, compliance and vital signs were assessed additionally at 8, 19, 32 and 45 weeks. PSA levels were measured at baseline and 52 weeks.

INCLUSION CRITERIA:
AUA-SS $\geq$ 8, PFR >4ml/s and <15ml/s, PVR urine $\leq$ 300ml.

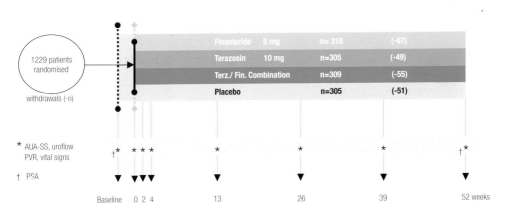

KEY RESULTS

- Terazosin and combination therapy were significantly effective compared to placebo in reducing AUA-SS at 12 months (reaching nadir at 13 weeks). Placebo 16.5%, finasteride 19.8%, terazosin 37.7% and combination 39%.

- Similarly, PFR was significantly increased in the terazosin (25.7%) and combination groups (30.1%) relative to placebo, reaching nadir at 4 weeks and being sustained at 12 months. Improvements in the placebo and finasteride groups were comparable (13.5% and 5.1%, respectively).

- Maximal changes in prostatic volume were significantly greater in the finasteride (↓16.9%) and combination groups (↓18.8%) than in the terazosin (↑1.3%) or placebo groups (↑1.3%).

- Dose reduction was required in 11% of patients in the terazosin and combination therapy groups and in 2% of patients in the finasteride and placebo groups.

- Withdrawals due to AEs were significantly lower in the placebo group than in all the other groups: placebo 1.6%, finasteride 4.8%, terazosin 5.9% and combination 7.8%.

Comparison of finasteride, terazosin and both combined in patients with BPH – efficacy outcomes after treatment for 12 months

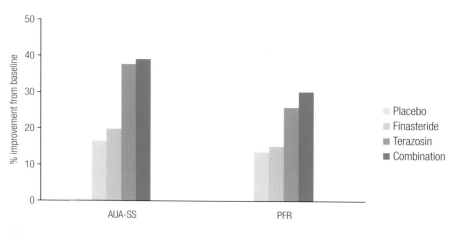

CONCLUSIONS FROM ORIGINAL REPORTS

Terazosin was an effective therapy in reducing the symptoms of BPH (symptom scores and urinary flow rate), whereas finasteride was not.
The combination of terazosin (10mg o.d.) and finasteride (5mg o.d.) was no more effective than terazosin alone.

POPULAR CITATION: Veterans Affairs Cooperative Study

STRENGTHS

This large, placebo-controlled, 4-arm study employed a variety of urodynamic and questionnaire-based endpoints.

WEAKNESSES

Only symptoms and urodynamic endpoints were evaluated. Additionally, this study only included patients with small prostate volumes. It could be argued that an effect on other endpoints (retention and surgery) could have been missed. It has been suggested that the duration   (1 year) was insufficient to show real benefit of finasteride.

RELEVANCE

This study is highly representative of the way in which α-blockers and finasteride could be used in combination in clinical practice. The alternative use of removing the α-blocker component from the combination is currently under evaluation.

An attempt to quantify the benefit of phytotherapy: Phytotherapy compared to finasteride in the treatment of benign prostatic hyperplasia.

KEY TRIAL REFERENCES

MAJOR PUBLICATION:
Carrraro J-C, Raynaud et al. Comparison of phytotherapy (Permixon®) with finasteride in the treatment of benign prostate hyperplasia: A randomised international study of 1,098 patients. Prostate 29:231-240, 1996.

ORIGINAL ABSTRACT: not published at AUA and EAU

OTHER IMPORTANT PUBLICATIONS:
Wilt T, Ishani A et al. Serenoa repens for benign prostatic hyperplasia. Cochrane Database Syst Rev 2:CD001423, 2000.

Boyle P, Robertson C et al. Meta-analysis of clinical trials of Permixon in the treatment of symptomatic benign prostatic hyperplasia. Urology 55(4):533-539, 2000.

STUDY FUNDING: Pierre Fabre Médicament

IMPORTANCE OF STUDY

This is one of the few controlled studies that have been completed on phytotherapy using validated, clinical endpoints.
The data purport to show that phytotherapy produces clinical benefit equivalent to finasteride.

Study Design

Double-blind, randomised, equivalence, multicentre study. n=1098.
Following baseline evaluations patients were randomised to either Permixon (160mg b.i.d.) or finasteride (5mg o.d.) for 6 months treatment.

Outcome measures:

IPSS (0-35 points), QoL score (0-6 points), sexual function score (0-20 points), PFR and mean flow rate were evaluated at baseline, 6, 13 and 26 weeks. Prostate volume, PVR and PSA were determined at baseline, 13 and 26 weeks.

Inclusion criteria:

IPSS >6, enlarged prostate on DRE, prostate volume >25ml, PFR 4-15ml/s, PSA <10ng/ml for prostates ≤ 60ml and <15ng/ml for prostates > 60ml.

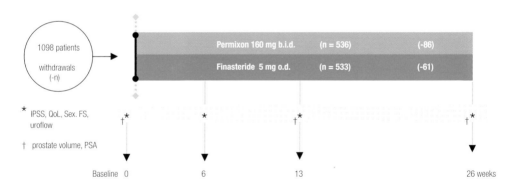

1098 patients
withdrawals
(-n)

Permixon 160 mg b.i.d. (n = 536) (-86)
Finasteride 5 mg o.d. (n = 533) (-61)

* IPSS, QoL, Sex. FS, uroflow

† prostate volume, PSA

Baseline 0   6   13   26 weeks

KEY RESULTS

- IPSSs were decreased in both groups at 26 weeks: Permixon (37%) and finasteride (39%).

- QoL scores were also improved with both treatments: Permixon (38%) and finasteride (41%).

- There were no statistical differences in the responses obtained with either drug for symptom scores or QoL scores.

- Sexual function scores deteriorated significantly with finasteride (+9%) compared to Permixon (−6%).

- PFR was increased in both groups at 26 weeks with finasteride giving superior results; Permixon (25%) and finasteride (30%) [$P=0.035$]. However, both treatments were comparable for the numbers of patients achieving a > 3ml/s increase in PFR: Permixon 36% and finasteride 39%.

- Prostate volume decreased significantly with finasteride (−18%) but not with Permixon (−6%).

- Serum PSA decreased significantly with finasteride (−41%) but increased slightly with Permixon (+3%)

- There were no statistically significant differences between the treatment groups in the incidence of any of the adverse events.

Comparison of finasteride and phytotherapy (Permixon) in the treatment of mild to moderate BPH – efficacy over 6 months

CONCLUSIONS FROM ORIGINAL REPORTS

Both Permixon and finasteride were clinically equivalent in patients with mild to moderate BPH and relieved the symptoms in about two thirds of patients.
Unlike finasteride, Permixon had no effect on androgen-dependent parameters, suggesting other pathways may be involved in the symptomatology of BPH.

POPULAR CITATION: not applicable

STRENGTHS

An active drug (finasteride)-controlled study using a wide variety of objective and subjective clinical endpoints.

WEAKNESSES

No placebo comparator was used in this study.
The time period used (26 weeks) was relatively short for finasteride to show its full efficacy.

RELEVANCE

On the assumption that finasteride is effective, Permixon could be considered to be equally so. However, the absence of a placebo arm should result in some caution with this interpretation. Changes seen for both finasteride and Permixon are comparable to the placebo response seen in other clinical trials.

STUDY DESCRIPTOR

This study is of great importance in calculation of healthcare costs for managing BPH patients: Transurethral surgery versus watchful waiting for the treatment of moderate symptoms of benign prostatic hyperplasia.

KEY TRIAL REFERENCES

MAJOR PUBLICATION:
Wasson J, Reda D et al. A comparison of transurethral surgery with watchful waiting for moderate symptoms of benign prostatic hyperplasia. N Engl J Med 332:75-79, 1995.

ORIGINAL ABSTRACT: not published at AUA or EAU

OTHER IMPORTANT PUBLICATIONS:
Bruskewitz R, Reda D et al. Testing to predict outcome after transurethral resection of the prostate. J Urol 157(4):1304-1308, 1997.

Flannigan R, Reda D et al. 5-year outcome of surgical resection and watchful waiting for men with moderately symptomatic benign prostatic hyperplasia: A Department of Veterans Affairs Cooperative Study. J Urol 160(1):12-16, 1998.

STUDY FUNDING: Veterans Affairs Medical Research Service

IMPORTANCE OF STUDY

The potential importance of this study is that it attempts to quantify the benefit of watchful waiting.
It shows that watchful waiting is safe in men with moderate LUTS. However, perhaps, not surprisingly watchful waiting is found to be of less benefit than surgery in terms of symptom relief or other clinical outcomes (e.g. treatment failure).

STUDY DESIGN

Randomised, multicentre, long-term study. n=556.
Following baseline evaluations patients were randomised to either surgery (n=280) or watchful waiting (ww) (n=276). Surgical patients underwent surgery within 2 weeks of randomisation. All patients were followed for 3 years.

OUTCOME MEASURES:
Primary outcome measure was treatment failure, defined as: death, repeated/ intractable urinary retention, PVR urine >350ml, bladder calculus, new/persistent incontinence, high symptom score (>24) or a doubling of serum creatinine. PFR, PVR urine, voided volume and symptoms were assessed at baseline and 6-monthly. QoL was assessed at baseline and annually.

INCLUSION CRITERIA:
>55 years, moderate to severe symptoms (10-20 points on a 27-point scale), PVR urine <350ml, serum creatinine >265mmol/l.

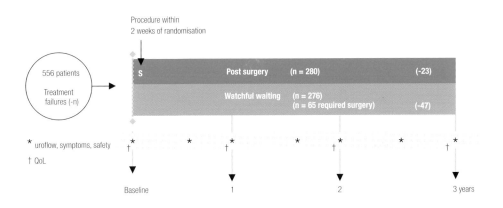

KEY RESULTS

- There were 23 treatment failures (3/100 person years) in the surgery group compared to 47 in the watchful waiting group (6.1/100 person years) over the 3 years. The higher rate in the ww group was mainly due to intractable urinary retention, large PVR urine and high symptom scores.

- In the ww group 65 men (24%) underwent surgery within the 3 years, 20 of them due to treatment failure.

- Surgery was associated with significant improvements in symptom score (66% vs 38%), QoL bother score (67% vs 20%), increase in PFR (55% vs 3%) and decrease in PVR urine (54% vs 36%).

- Surgery was also associated with a higher detection rate for prostate cancer, 9.6% vs 2.9% in the ww group.

- For men in the ww group the rate of crossover to surgery was twice as high for those who had high baseline scores for bother from urinary symptoms.

Surgery versus watchful waiting for men with moderate symptoms of BPH – treatment outcomes after 3 years follow-up

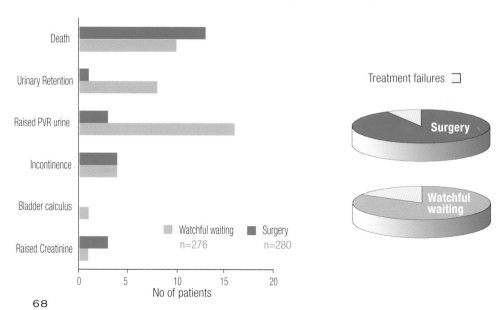

CONCLUSIONS FROM ORIGINAL REPORTS

Surgery is more effective in reducing treatment failure and improving urinary symptoms than watchful waiting for men with moderate symptoms of BPH.
Watchful waiting is usually a safe alternative for those men who are less bothered by urinary symptoms, or who wish to delay surgery.

POPULAR CITATION: not applicable

STRENGTHS

This is a prospective, parallel arm study using a relatively large number of patients.

WEAKNESSES

For ethical reasons, patients with severe symptoms were excluded. There were no evaluations in patients with mild symptoms at baseline (presumably as surgery would not be an option).

RELEVANCE

This study is reassuring in so far as watchful waiting is likely to be safe and could be of some benefit in a patient sub-population who might otherwise be scheduled for surgery.

STUDY DESCRIPTOR

Trial of significance beyond BPH that describes the steps necessary for questionnaire development and validation: The American Urological Association Symptom Index for benign prostatic hyperplasia.

KEY TRIAL REFERENCES

MAJOR PUBLICATION:
Barry M, Fowler F et al. The American Urological Association Symptom Index for benign prostatic hyperplasia. J Urol 148:1549-1557, 1992.

OTHER IMPORTANT PUBLICATIONS:
Barry M, Fowler F et al. Correlation of the American Urological Association Symptom index with self-administered versions of the Madsen-Iversen, Boyarsky and Maine Medical Assessment Program symptom indexes. Measurement Committee of the American Urological Association. J Urol 148(5):1558-1563, 1992.

Barry M, Fowler F et al. The American Urological Association Symptom Index: does mode of administration affect its psychometric properties? J Urol 154(3):1056-1059.

Barry M, Williford W et al. Benign prostatic hyperplasia specific health status measures in clinical research: how much change in the American Urological Association Symptom Index and Benign Prostatic Hyperplasia Impact index is perceptible to patients? J Urol 154(5):1770-1774, 1995.

STUDY FUNDING: Agency of Health Care Policy and Research American Urological Association

IMPORTANCE OF STUDY

The value of this study goes beyond BPH clinical trial methodology. This trial exemplifies the rigour required in the development and validation of a questionnaire-based scoring system.

Prior to the development of the AUA symptom index there was no objective and reliable means (apart from urodynamics) for either clinical diagnosis or determination of drug effects. This trial shows the development process for a standardised, reliable and self-administered questionnaire.

STUDY DESIGN

Validation study. n=210 BPH patients and 108 control subjects.

INCLUSION CRITERIA:

For BPH patients, clinical diagnosis of BPH. For control subjects, 18-55 years and no urinary complaints.

FIRST VALIDATION STUDY:

A 15-item questionnaire was developed by members of the Measurement Committee of the AUA, covering the domains of daytime frequency, nocturia, hesitancy, intermittency, weak stream, incomplete emptying, terminal dribbling and dysuria. Additionally 2 global questions relating to bothersomeness were posed. This questionnaire was self-administered to BPH patients (n=76) and control subjects (n=59), initially in the office setting and then again 1 week later by mail. The responses to this questionnaire were analysed in terms of difficulty experienced in answering, distribution of answers across the response frame and for correlation to the global problem questions. Test-retest reliabilities were also analysed.

From the analysis of responses to the 15-item questionnaire 6 questions were selected covering emptying, frequency, intermittency, urgency, weak stream and nocturia to create the AUA-6 index. Subsequently a question on hesitancy was added to form the AUA-7 index, although there had been modest correlation with the global bother question and the questions in AUA-6, hesitancy is regarded as a classic symptom of BPH.

SECOND VALIDATION STUDY:

The AUA-6 and AUA-7 indices were administered to another 107 BPH patients and 49 control subjects in a similar manner to that used in the first study.

RESPONSIVENESS STUDY:

The AUA-7 index was administered pre-operatively and 4 weeks post-operatively to 27 patients undergoing either transurethral or open prostatectomy.

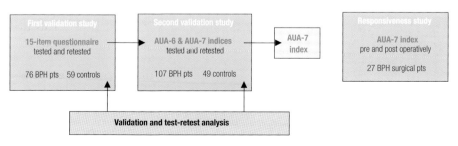

KEY RESULTS

- The final AUA symptom index includes 7 questions covering frequency, nocturia, weak urinary stream, hesitancy, intermittence, incomplete emptying and urgency. Each question was scored 0-5, with 5 being most severe, giving a total score range of 0-35.

- On revalidation the index was internally consistent and had excellent test-retest reliability (r=0.92).

- Scores were highly correlated to subjects' global ratings of the magnitude of their urinary problem (r=0.65 to 0.72).

- The scores for this index also powerfully discriminated between BPH patients and control subjects.

- In the responsiveness study the index was sensitive to change, with preoperative scores decreasing from a mean of 17.6 to 7.1 by 4 weeks post surgery (p<0.001).

AUA symptom index
– distribution of answers amongst BPH patients and controls

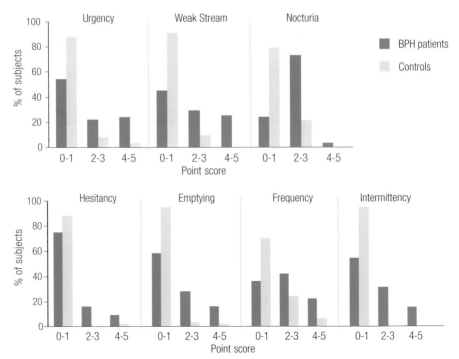

CONCLUSIONS FROM ORIGINAL REPORTS

This self-administered AUA symptom index is a reliable and valid method of capturing the symptom severity of clinically defined BPH.

The scores of this index are sensitive to clinically important changes for individual patients over time.

These features are desirable in a questionnaire that may also be used for predictive, discriminative or evaluative purposes.

POPULAR CITATION: not applicable

STRENGTHS

This scoring system was developed by world-class experts.

The system was statistically validated and adequately powered in BPH patients and controls.

WEAKNESSES

No active agent was included, therefore sensitivity to change resulting from pharmacological intervention was not analysed by this trial.

RELEVANCE

This is a model of good clinical trial design for BPH studies.

Inclusion and exclusion criteria are such that the study population is likely to be representative of the BPH patient 'at large'.

Key trial attempting to quantify the placebo effect observed in all BPH studies: Placebo therapy for benign prostatic hyperplasia.

KEY TRIAL REFERENCES

MAJOR PUBLICATION:
Nickel J for the Canadian PROSPECT Study Group. Placebo therapy of benign prostatic hyperplasia: a 25-month study. Br J Urol 81:383-387, 1998.

ORIGINAL ABSTRACT:
Societe Internationale d'Urologie 24th World Congress, Montreal, Sept. 7-11, 1997.

FIRST PUBLICATION:
Nickel J, Fradet Y et al. Efficacy and safety of finasteride therapy for benign prostatic hyperplasia: results of a 2-year randomised controlled trial (the PROSPECT study). PROscar Safety Plus Efficacy Canadian Two year study. CMAJ 155(9):1251-1259, 1996.

STUDY FUNDING: Merck & Co

IMPORTANCE OF STUDY

An unequivocal evaluation of the long-term placebo effect in one clinical trial. This study exemplifies the need for a placebo control in BPH trials. Previous attempts at quantification of the placebo effect have been misleading, as any response would be diluted by a placebo run-in incorporated in the design.

STUDY DESIGN

Randomised, double-blind, placebo-controlled, long-term, multicentre study. n=303.
This study analyses the placebo arm of the PROSPECT study that compared long-term finasteride therapy with placebo. All patients underwent 1-month placebo run-in before randomisation to 2 years further treatment.

OUTCOME MEASURES:
Boyarsky (modified) symptom scores and PFR were assessed at baseline, 1 month and every 4 months. Prostate volume was determined at baseline, 13 and 25 months. Adverse events (including occurrence of AUR and surgery).

INCLUSION CRITERIA:
<80 years, 2 moderate symptoms of BPH, (but no more than 2 severe symptoms), enlarged prostate on DRE, PFR 5-15ml/s, PVR urine <150ml, PSA <10ng/ml.

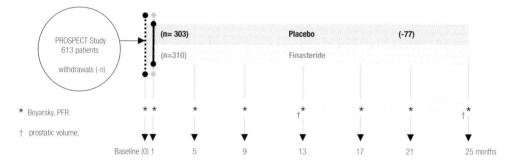

* Boyarsky, PFR

† prostatic volume,

KEY RESULTS

FOR PLACEBO PATIENTS:

- The mean total symptom score was significantly improved over baseline for the entire 25 months [p ≤ 0.001]. Total scores were improved by 2.9 points (16%) during the first 2 months and by 3.2 points (17%) at 9 months, the improvement declining to 2.3 (13%) at 25 months.

- Mean PFR improved from baseline by an average of 1.4ml/s (14%) over the first 5 months and remained improved by 1.0ml/s or more at 25 months.

- Prostate volume showed a progressive increase over the 25 months (+8.4%).

- The extent of the placebo response for symptom scores and PFR was independent of age but did correlate with initial symptom severity and PFR. Patients with a prostate volume ≤ 40ml had a clinically more important placebo response than those with larger prostates.

- Adverse events thought to be secondary to placebo treatment were reported by 81% of patients. The most common AEs were urogenital (40%), specifically impotence (6.3%) and decreased libido (6.3%). Withdrawals due to significant AEs were 13.2%. AUR was experienced by 3.3% of patients and 8.6% of the group required a urological surgical intervention.

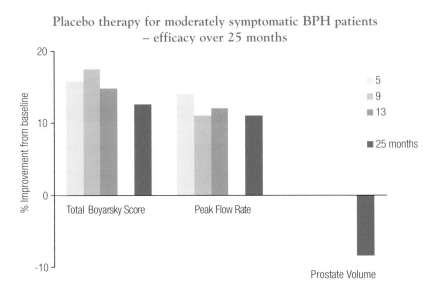

Placebo therapy for moderately symptomatic BPH patients – efficacy over 25 months

CONCLUSIONS FROM ORIGINAL REPORTS

For patients with moderately symptomatic BPH, placebo therapy produced a rapid and significant improvement in urinary symptoms and uroflow. Although the beneficial effects fade they are still present after 2 years placebo treatment.
Placebo therapy is also associated with clinically important adverse effects.
For the accurate evaluation of the potential benefits of any intervention for symptomatic BPH, long-term placebo (or sham-control) clinical trials are required and should be of > 2 years in duration.

POPULAR CITATION: PROSPECT (Proscar Safety Plus Efficacy Canadian Two-year study)

STRENGTHS

An adequately powered study using several relevant questionnaire-based and urological endpoints.

WEAKNESSES

Only a sub-population of moderately symptomatic BPH patients was followed. Placebo response could be different in patients with mild or severe symptomatology.

RELEVANCE

The improvements in symptoms and urodynamics are likely to be predictive of the clinical placebo response in BPH patients and/or the impact of watchful waiting. However, this is not representative of normal clinical trial design.

STUDY DESCRIPTOR

Important trial defining the underlying basis of placebo effect and giving insight into better trial design: Analysis of the 'placebo effect' in benign prostatic hyperplasia treatment trials.

KEY TRIAL REFERENCES

MAJOR PUBLICATION:
Sech S, Montoya J et al. The so-called 'placebo effect' in benign prostatic hyperplasia treatment trials represents partially a conditional regression to the mean induced by censoring. Urology 51:242-250, 1998.

ORIGINAL ABSTRACT: not published at AUA and EAU

OTHER IMPORTANT PUBLICATIONS:
Barnboym E, Ahrens A, Roehrborn C. Effect of scrambling on short-term reliability of the American Urological Association Symptom Index. Urology 53(3):568-573, 1999.

Roehrborn C, Malice M et al. Clinical predictors of spontaneous acute urinary retention in men with LUTS and clinical BPH: a comprehensive analysis of the pooled groups of several large clinical trials. Urology 58(2):210-216, 2001.

STUDY FUNDING:

IMPORTANCE OF STUDY

This study is the first comprehensive analysis of the components of the 'placebo' response in BPH patients. The trial shows that as a result of inclusion and exclusion criteria there will be a natural regression to the mean, irrespective of any drug effect. This 'effect' also complicates the interpretation of the data.

Study Design

Double-blind, analysis of clinical trial methodology. n=145.
Volunteers were asked to complete an AUA symptom index, BPH impact index, QoL score and perform a urinary flow rate test. The subjects completed the same assessments 2 weeks later. Subjects received no consultation from physician, no therapeutic intervention and no indication of the nature or purpose of the study. Complete sets of data were obtained for both sets of assessments.

Typical BPH selection criteria were applied to the first set of results (AUA score of 7, 10, 12 or 15 points, PFR of <15, <12, <10 ml/s) and these qualifying subjects progressed to have their second test results included in the second test analysis. Similar criteria were applied to the BPH-II scores.

INCLUSION CRITERIA: Male volunteers with no known urological conditions.

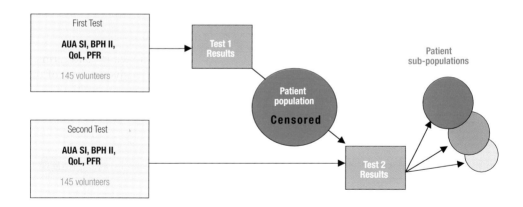

KEY RESULTS

■ There was good correlation between the 2 sets of test results (AUA SI, BPH II, QoL and PFR) with correlation coefficients between 0.73 and 0.89, when all subjects were considered. The small changes in the means between the 2 sets of tests tended to be improvement for AUA SI, BPH II and QoL and a decrease for PFR.

■ Censoring subjects and their exclusion from the analysis of the second test induced a regression to the mean phenomenon, resulting in an artificial improvement in these outcome parameters.

■ The magnitude of the improvements increased when tighter selection and censoring criteria were applied.

Effect of censoring on efficacy outcome parameters.
Application of increasingly tighter selection criteria increases the magnitude of improvement
(Tests conducted in 145 untreated volunteers with no known urological disease)

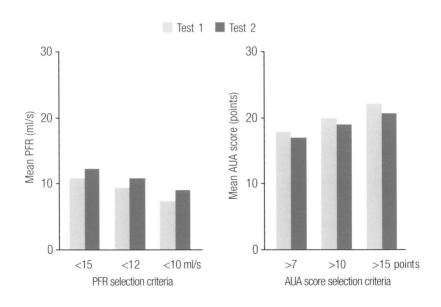

CONCLUSIONS FROM ORIGINAL REPORTS

Censoring of patients by application of inclusion and exclusion criteria is typical of BPH trials. The effect of this censoring is a regression to the mean, which leads to an apparent improvement in outcome parameters.

POPULAR CITATION: not applicable

STRENGTHS

A wide variety of parameters covering, symptoms, urodynamics and QoL were employed.

WEAKNESSES

Only 2 sets of measurements were made in each patient.

RELEVANCE

This is a powerful message that relates to clinical trial design (powering, inclusion, exclusion criteria). However, this does not relate to clinical management of BPH patients.